World Health Organization

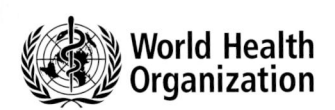

GUIDELINES
ON HEPATITIS B AND C TESTING

FEBRUARY 2017

GUIDELINES

WHO guidelines on hepatitis B and C testing

ISBN 978-92-4-154998-1

© World Health Organization 2017

Some rights reserved. This work is available under the Creative Commons Attribution-NonCommercial-ShareAlike 3.0 IGO licence (CC BY-NC-SA 3.0 IGO; https://creativecommons.org/licenses/by-nc-sa/3.0/igo).

Under the terms of this licence, you may copy, redistribute and adapt the work for non-commercial purposes, provided the work is appropriately cited, as indicated below. In any use of this work, there should be no suggestion that WHO endorses any specific organization, products or services. The use of the WHO logo is not permitted. If you adapt the work, then you must license your work under the same or equivalent Creative Commons licence. If you create a translation of this work, you should add the following disclaimer along with the suggested citation: "This translation was not created by the World Health Organization (WHO). WHO is not responsible for the content or accuracy of this translation. The original English edition shall be the binding and authentic edition".

Any mediation relating to disputes arising under the licence shall be conducted in accordance with the mediation rules of the World Intellectual Property Organization.

Suggested citation. WHO guidelines on hepatitis B and C testing. Geneva: World Health Organization; 2017. Licence: CC BY-NC-SA 3.0 IGO.

Cataloguing-in-Publication (CIP) data. CIP data are available at http://apps.who.int/iris.

Sales, rights and licensing. To purchase WHO publications, see http://apps.who.int/bookorders. To submit requests for commercial use and queries on rights and licensing, see http://www.who.int/about/licensing.

Third-party materials. If you wish to reuse material from this work that is attributed to a third party, such as tables, figures or images, it is your responsibility to determine whether permission is needed for that reuse and to obtain permission from the copyright holder. The risk of claims resulting from infringement of any third-party-owned component in the work rests solely with the user.

General disclaimers. The designations employed and the presentation of the material in this publication do not imply the expression of any opinion whatsoever on the part of WHO concerning the legal status of any country, territory, city or area or of its authorities, or concerning the delimitation of its frontiers or boundaries. Dotted and dashed lines on maps represent approximate border lines for which there may not yet be full agreement.

The mention of specific companies or of certain manufacturers' products does not imply that they are endorsed or recommended by WHO in preference to others of a similar nature that are not mentioned. Errors and omissions excepted, the names of proprietary products are distinguished by initial capital letters.

All reasonable precautions have been taken by WHO to verify the information contained in this publication. However, the published material is being distributed without warranty of any kind, either expressed or implied. The responsibility for the interpretation and use of the material lies with the reader. In no event shall WHO be liable for damages arising from its use.

Printed in China

Design and layout: blossoming.it

CONTENTS

ACKNOWLEDGEMENTS	x
ABBREVIATIONS AND ACRONYMS	xiv
GLOSSARY OF TERMS	xvi
EXECUTIVE SUMMARY	xxi
SUMMARY ALGORITHMS	xxvi
SUMMARY OF RECOMMENDATIONS	xxvii

PART 1: BACKGROUND — 1

1. INTRODUCTION — 2
- 1.1. Current challenges in viral hepatitis testing — 2
- 1.2. Goals of viral hepatitis testing — 3
- 1.3. Why are testing guidelines needed? — 4
- 1.4. Goals and objectives of the guidelines — 5
- 1.5. Scope of the guidelines — 5
- 1.6. Target audience — 6
- 1.7. Related WHO materials and guidelines — 6

2. GUIDING PRINCIPLES — 8
- 2.1. Promoting human rights and equity in access to hepatitis testing — 8
- 2.2. The public health approach along the continuum of care — 8
- 2.3. The WHO "5 Cs" — 9
- 2.4. Accurate testing — 9

3. METHODOLOGY AND PROCESS OF DEVELOPING THE GUIDELINES — 10
- 3.1. WHO guideline development process — 10
- 3.2. Systematic reviews and additional background work — 10
- 3.3. Grading of quality of evidence and strength of recommendations — 11
- 3.4. Formulation of recommendations — 14
- 3.5. Declaration and management of conflicts of interest — 15
- 3.6. Updating, disseminating and monitoring implementation of the guidelines — 15

4. BACKGROUND – EPIDEMIOLOGY AND NATURAL HISTORY — 16
- 4.1. **Hepatitis B infection** — 19
  - 4.1.1. Epidemiology of hepatitis B infection — 19
  - 4.1.2. Transmission of hepatitis B infection — 20
  - 4.1.3. Natural history of HBV infection — 20
  - 4.1.4. Time course and interpretation of serological markers of HBV infection — 21
  - 4.1.5. Preventing hepatitis B infection through vaccination — 24
  - 4.1.6. Treatment of hepatitis B infection — 24

4.2.	**Hepatitis C infection**	24
4.2.1.	Epidemiology of hepatitis C infection	24
4.2.2.	Transmission of hepatitis C infection	25
4.2.3.	Natural history of hepatitis C infection	27
4.2.4.	Time course of serological markers for HCV infection	27
4.2.5.	Prevention of hepatitis C infection	28
4.2.6.	Treatment of hepatitis C infection	28

5. BACKGROUND – DIAGNOSTICS FOR TESTING FOR HEPATITIS B AND C INFECTION — 30

5.1.	Types of viral hepatitis assays	30
5.2	Serological assays	30
5.3.	Nucleic acid testing (NAT) technologies	31
5.4.	Choice of serological assays	32
5.5.	Selection of a one or two assay serological testing strategy	32

PART 2: RECOMMENDATIONS — 35

6. WHO TO TEST FOR CHRONIC HEPATITIS B OR C INFECTION
– testing approaches and service delivery — 36

6.1.	Recommendations	36
6.2.	Background	38

6A TESTING APPROACHES TO DETECT CHRONIC HEPATITIS B — 40

6.3.	Summary of the evidence	40
6.4.	Rationale for the recommendations	41

6B TESTING APPROACHES TO DETECT CHRONIC HEPATITIS C — 45

6.5.	Summary of the evidence	45
6.6.	Rationale for the recommendations	46

6C SERVICE DELIVERY OF HEPATITIS B AND C TESTING — 49

6.7.	Rationale for the recommendations on community-based testing	49
6.8.	Rationale for the recommendations on facility-based testing	50
6.9.	Implementation considerations for HBV and HCV testing approaches	51

7. HOW TO TEST FOR CHRONIC HEPATITIS B INFECTION
– choice of serological assay and testing strategy — 52

7.1.	Recommendations	52
7.2.	Background	53
7.3.	Summary of the evidence	54
7.4.	Rationale for the recommendations on which assay to use	57
7.5.	Rationale for the recommendations on testing strategy	59

8. HOW TO TEST FOR CURRENT OR PAST HCV INFECTION (HCV EXPOSURE) – choice of serological assay and testing strategy — 61
- 8.1. Recommendations — 61
- 8.2. Background — 62
- 8.3. Summary of the evidence — 62
- 8.4. Rationale for the recommendations on which assay to use — 65
- 8.5. Rationale for the recommendation for a one-serological assay testing strategy — 67
- 8.6. Implementation considerations for HBsAg and HCV antibody serological testing — 68

9. DETECTION OF VIRAEMIC HBV INFECTION – to guide who to treat or not treat — 70
- 9.1. Recommendation — 70
- 9.2. Background — 72
- 9.3. Rationale for the recommendations (WHO 2015 HBV guidelines) — 72
- 9.4. Implementation considerations — 73

10. MONITORING FOR HBV TREATMENT RESPONSE AND DISEASE PROGRESSION — 74
- 10.1. Recommendations — 74
- 10.2. Background – goals of monitoring — 74
- 10.3. Rationale for the recommendations (WHO 2015 HBV guidelines) — 75
- 10.4. Implementation considerations — 76

11. DETECTION OF VIRAEMIC HCV INFECTION – to guide who to treat — 77
- 11.1. Recommendations — 77
- 11.2. Background — 77
- 11.3. Summary of the evidence — 78
- 11.4. Rationale for the recommendations — 80
- 11.5. Implementation considerations — 81

12. ASSESSMENT OF HCV TREATMENT RESPONSE — 83
- 12.1. Recommendation — 83
- 12.2. Background — 83
- 12.3. Summary of the evidence — 83
- 12.4. Rationale for the recommendations — 84
- 12.5. Implementation considerations — 85

13. USE OF DRIED BLOOD SPOT SPECIMENS FOR SEROLOGICAL AND VIROLOGICAL TESTING — 86
- 13.1. Recommendations — 86
- 13.2. Background — 86
- 13.3. Summary of the evidence — 87
- 13.4. Rationale for the recommendations — 89
- 13.5. Implementation considerations — 92

14. IMPROVING THE UPTAKE OF TESTING AND LINKAGE TO CARE AND PREVENTION — 95
- 14.1. Recommendations — 95
- 14.2. Background — 95
- 14.3. Summary of the evidence — 96
- 14.4. Rationale for the recommendations — 98
- 14.5. Implementation considerations — 100

PART 3: IMPLEMENTATION — 101

15. IMPLEMENTING LABORATORY TESTING SERVICES FOR VIRAL HEPATITIS — 102
- 15.1. Key elements for national testing services — 102
- 15.2. National framework for viral hepatitis testing — 103
- 15.3. Building capacity for testing services — 104
- 15.4. Product selection — 106
- 15.5. Assuring the quality of testing services — 109
- 15.6. Assuring the safety of testing services — 111
- 15.7. Other practical considerations for testing — 111

16. PRE-TEST AND POST-TEST COUNSELLING — 114
- 16.1. Promoting testing awareness — 114
- 16.2. Creating an enabling environment — 115
- 16.3. The WHO 5 "Cs" — 115
- 16.4. Providing pre-test information — 116
- 16.5. Post-test counseling and services — 117

17. SERVICE DELIVERY APPROACHES TO VIRAL HEPATITIS TESTING – examples from the field — 119
- 17.1. Health-care facility-based testing — 120
- 17.2. Community-based testing — 123
- 17.3. Good practices for delivery of effective viral hepatitis testing services — 127
- 17.4. Diagnostic innovations to promote access to testing — 130

18. TESTING ISSUES IN SPECIFIC POPULATIONS — 132
- 18.1 Principles for testing in all populations — 132
- 18.2 Principles for testing in key populations — 132
- 18.3. Persons living with HIV — 135
- 18.4. Tuberculosis-infected populations — 135
- 18.5. Migrant and mobile populations — 136
- 18.6. Health-care workers — 136
- 18.7. Couples, partners, family members and household contacts — 137
- 18.8. Pregnant women — 138
- 18.9. Children — 139
- 18.10. Adolescents — 141

19. STRATEGIC PLANNING FOR IMPLEMENTING TESTING SERVICES AND APPROACHES   143

Step 1: Review national and subnational epidemiology   146
Step 2: Set testing (and treatment) coverage targets   147
Step 3: Review the effectiveness of and identify gaps in hepatitis testing service delivery   147
Step 4: Assess costs and review cost–effectiveness of different testing approaches   149
Step 5: Adjust programmes and monitor   150

REFERENCES   152

Web annexes

All annexes will be available on the WHO hepatitis website.

Annex 1: The Global Hepatitis Health Sector Strategy – global targets

Annex 2: Guidelines for the prevention, care and treatment of persons with chronic hepatitis B infection – summary of recommendations

Annex 3: Guidelines for the screening, care and treatment of persons with chronic hepatitis C infection – summary of recommendations

Annex 4: PICO questions and decision-making tables

Annex 5: Systematic reviews and evidence summaries

Annex 6: Predictive modelling analysis

Annex 7: Summary of declared interests

Annex 8: Systematic review teams, Guideline Steering Group, Guideline Development Group, External Review Group

ACKNOWLEDGEMENTS

Many professionals from a range of backgrounds and specialties have contributed to the development of this guidance. WHO is sincerely grateful for their time and support.

Guidelines Development Group

The chair of the Guidelines Development Group was Margaret Hellard (Burnet Institute, Melbourne Australia). Roger Chou (Oregon Health and Science University, Portland, USA) was the guidelines methodologist.

The following experts served on the Guidelines Development Group:

Jacinto Amandua (Ministry of Health, Uganda); Isabelle Andrieux-Meyer (Médecins Sans Frontières, Geneva, Switzerland); Manal Hamdy El-Sayed (Egypt National Hepatitis Committee, Cairo, Egypt); Charles Gore (World Hepatitis Alliance, London, UK); Niklas Luhmann (Médicins du Monde, Paris, France); Michael Ninburg (Hepatitis Education Project, Seattle, USA); Richard Njouom (Centre Pasteur, Cameroon); John Parry (Public Health England, London, UK); Trevor Peter (Clinton Health Access Initiative, New York, USA); Teri Roberts (Foundation for Innovative New Diagnostics, Geneva, Switzerland); Giten Khwairakpam Singh (TREAT Asia/amFAR, Bangkok, Thailand); Lara Tavoschi (European Center for Disease Prevention and Control, Stockholm, Sweden); Richard Tedder – unable to attend (Public Health England, London, UK).

WHO regions: Fabian Ndenzako (WHO Regional Office for Africa), Nicole Simone Seguy (WHO Country Office, India), Nick Walsh (WHO Regional Office for the Western Pacific).

Contributors to the systematic reviews

We would like to credit the following researchers for conducting the systematic reviews, evidence profiles and GRADE tables: Ali Amini (London School of Hygiene and Tropical Medicine, London, UK); Debra Boeras (London School of Hygiene and Tropical Medicine, London, UK); Wen Chen (London School of Hygiene and Tropical Medicine, London, UK); Jennifer Cohn (Médecins Sans Frontières, Geneva, Switzerland – Team leader); Claudia Denkinger (Foundation for Innovative New Diagnostics, Geneva, Switzerland – Team leader); Jane Falconer (London School of Hygiene and Tropical Medicine, London, UK); Thomas Fitzpatrick (University of Washington, School of Medicine, Seattle, USA – Team leader); Timothy Hallet

(Imperial College, London, UK – Team leader); Helen Kelly (London School of Hygiene and Tropical Medicine, London, UK); Mellanye Lackey (University of Utah, Salt Lake City, USA); Berit Lange (University Hospital, Freiburg, Germany); Ying-Ru Lo (WHO Regional Office for the Western Pacific); Shevanthi Nayagam (Imperial College, London, UK); Rosanna Peeling (London School of Hygiene and Tropical Medicine, London, UK – Team leader); Teri Roberts (Foundation for Innovative New Diagnostics, Geneva, Switzerland); Julia Scott (WHO Regional Office for the Western Pacific); Weiming Tang (London School of Hygiene and Tropical Medicine, London, UK); Edouard Tuaillon (Montpellier Teaching Hospital, France); Joseph Tucker (UNC Project-China, University of North Carolina, USA – Team leader); Philippe Van de Perre (Université Montpellier, Montpellier, France); Olivia Varsaneux (London School of Hygiene and Tropical Medicine, London, UK); Nick Walsh (WHO Regional Office for the Western Pacific); Ji Young Kim (WHO Regional Office for the Western Pacific); Kali Zhou (University of California, Department of Medicine, San Francisco, USA – Team leader).

Contributors to supporting evidence

Predictive modelling: Benjamin Linas (Boston University School of Medicine, Boston, USA – Team leader); Jake Morgan (Boston University School of Medicine, Boston, USA); John Parry (Public Health England, London, UK).
Values and preferences survey: Elena Ivanova, Teri Roberts, and Alessandra Trianni (Foundation for Innovative New Diagnostics, Geneva, Switzerland).
Feasibility survey: Julie Bouscaillou and Niklas Luhmann (Médicins du Monde, Paris, France); Philippa Easterbrook and Azumi Ishizaki (WHO headquarters).
Case studies: John Best (University of California, San Francisco, USA); Kathrine Myers (Aaron Diamond AIDS Research Center, USA); and Joseph Tucker (University of North Carolina, and the International Diagnostics Centre, China).

External peer review group

The following experts served as external peer reviewers of the draft guidelines:

Tanya Applegate (Kirby Institute, Australia); Susan Best (National Serology Reference Laboratory, Australia); Yap Boum (Epicentre, Medecins sans Frontière, France); Alaa Gad Hashish (Al Shams University, Egypt); Joumana Hermez (WHO, Egypt); Cami Graham (Beth Israel Deaconess Medical Center, USA); Stephen Locarnini (Doherty Institute, Australia); Jean-Bosco Ndinokubwayo (WHO Regional Office for Africa); Ponsiano Ocama (Makerere University, Uganda); Jilian Sacks (Clinton Health Access Initiative, USA); Jules Mugabo Semahore (WHO, Rwanda); Mark Sonderup (University of Cape Town, South Africa); Gilles Wandeler (University of Bern, Swizerland).

Hepatitis testing innovation contest: Steering Group: Joseph Tucker (University of North Carolina, SESH, and the International Diagnostics Centre, China), Kathrine Myers (Aaron Diamond AIDS Research Center, USA), John Best (University of California, San Francisco, USA), and Philippa Easterbrook (Global Hepatitis Programme, WHO HQ, Switzerland).

Judging panel: Isabelle Andrieux-Meyer (Médecins Sans Frontières, Switzerland); Betty Apica (Makerere University College of Health Sciences, Uganda); Tasnim Azim (International Centre for Diarrhoeal Disease Research, Bangladesh); Carmen Figueroa (WHO, Switzerland); Charles Gore (Hepatitis C Trust and World Hepatitis Alliance, United Kingdom); Azumi Ishizaki (WHO, Switzerland); Kenneth Kabagambe (The National Organisation for People Living with Hepatitis B Uganda); Karyn Kaplan (Treatment Action Group, USA); Medhi Karkouri (Association de Lutte Contre le Sida, Morocco); Giten Khwairakpam Singh (TREAT Asia/amfAR, Thailand); Othman Mellouk (ITPC Global); Veronica Miller (Forum for Collaborative HIV Research, USA); Antons Mozalevskis (WHO Regional Office for Europe, Copenhagen, Denmark); Michael Ninburg (Hepatitis Education Project, USA); Ponsiano Ocama (Makerere University, College of Health Sciences, Uganda); Rosanna Peeling (London School of Hygiene & Tropical Medicine and International Diagnostics Centre, United Kingdom); Razia Pendse (WHO Regional Office for South-East Asia, India); Gabriele Riedner (WHO Regional Office for the Eastern Mediterranean, Egypt); Patricia Velez (Guatemalan Liver Association); Nick Walsh (WHO Regional Office for the Western Pacific).

Steering Committee

The following WHO staff formed the Guidelines Steering Committee:

Rachel Baggaley (HIV Key Populations and Innovative Prevention); Cheryl Johnson (HIV Key Populations and Innovative Prevention); Anita Sands (Essential Medicines and Health Products), Willy Urassa (Essential Medicines and Health Products); Shaffiq Essajee (Treatment and Care, HIV/AIDS); Marco Vitoria (Treatment and Care, HIV/AIDS); Nicolas Campion Clark (Mental Health and Substance Abuse); Junping Yu (Blood and Transfusion Safety, Service Delivery and Safety).

Guidelines writing was led by Philippa Easterbrook (WHO headquarters), Surjo De and Sam Lattimore (Public Health England, University College London Hospital, London, UK); Elizabeth Peach (Melbourne, Australia); Anita Sands (WHO headquarters), and Jilian Sacks (Clinton Health Access Initiative [CHAI]). Drafts were reviewed and input provided by members of the Systematic Review teams, Guidelines Development Group, peer reviewers and WHO Secretariat staff.

We extend our gratitude to the following individuals of the WHO Secretariat and regional WHO offices for excellent support to the Steering Committee and the Guidelines Development Group:

Azumi Ishizaki, Judith van Holten, Sarah Hess, Marc Bulterys, Stefan Wiktor, Andrew Ball, Gottfried Hirnschall, Yvan Hutin, Hande Harmanci, Taner Jonathan Bertuna, Bandana Malhotra, Oyuntungalag Namjilsuren, Han Qin, Nick Walsh, Fabian Ndenzako, Nicole Simone Seguy.

Overall coordination

Philippa Easterbrook (Global Hepatitis Programme).

Funding

Funding for the development of these guidelines was provided by United States Centers for Disease Control and Prevention (CDC).

ABBREVIATIONS AND ACRONYMS

ALP	alkaline phosphatase
ALT	alanine aminotransferase
ANC	antenatal clinic
APRI	aminotransferase/platelet ratio index
ART	antiretroviral therapy
ARV	antiretroviral (drug)
AST	aspartate aminotransferase
CDC	U.S. Centers for Disease Control and Prevention
CG	Cockcroft–Gault
CHB	chronic hepatitis B
CI	confidence interval
CLIA	chemiluminescence immunoassay
CrCl	creatinine clearance
DAA	direct-acting antiviral (drug)
DALY	disability-adjusted life year
DBS	dried blood spot (specimen)
ECL	electrochemiluminescence immunoassay
eGFR	estimated glomerular filtration rate
EIA	enzyme immunoassay
ELISA	enzyme-linked immunosorbent assay
EQAS	external quality assessment scheme
FBC	full blood count
FDA	U.S. Food and Drug Administration
FIB-4	fibrosis-4 score
GDP	gross domestic product
gGT	gamma glutamyl transpeptidase
GHTF	Global Harmonization Task Force
GHSS	Global Health Sector Strategy
GRADE	Grading of Recommendations Assessment, Development and Evaluation
HBcAg	hepatitis B core antigen
HBeAg	hepatitis B e antigen
HBIG	hepatitis B immunoglobulin
HBsAg	hepatitis B surface antigen
HBV	hepatitis B virus
HCC	hepatocellular carcinoma
HCV	hepatitis C virus
HCVcAg	hepatitis C virus core antigen
HDV	hepatitis D virus
HIC	high-income country
HIV	human immunodeficiency virus
ICER	incremental cost–effectiveness ratio
IFN	interferon

IQR	interquartile range
IVD	in vitro diagnostic (medical device)
LMICs	low- and middle-income countries
LoD	limit of detection
LY	life year
M&E	monitoring and evaluation
MSM	men who have sex with men
MTCT	mother-to-child transmission
NAT	nucleic acid testing
NGO	nongovernmental organization
NIT	non-invasive test
NPV	negative predictive value
NRTI	nucleos(t)ide reverse transcriptase inhibitor
OR	odds ratio
OST	opioid substitution therapy
PCR	polymerase chain reaction
PEG-IFN	pegylated interferon
PICO	population, intervention, comparison, outcomes
PITC	provider-initiated testing and counselling
PMTCT	prevention of mother-to-child transmission
PPV	positive predictive value
PQ	(WHO) prequalification
PWID	people who inject drugs
QA	quality assurance
QALY	quality-adjusted life year
QC	quality control
QI	quality improvement
RBV	ribavirin
RCT	randomized controlled trial
RDT	rapid diagnostic test
RNA	ribonucleic acid
RR	relative risk
SOP	standard operating procedure
SSA	sub-Saharan Africa
STI	sexually transmitted infection
SVR	sustained virological response
TDF	tenofovir
ULN	upper limit of normal
UNAIDS	Joint United Nations Programme on HIV/AIDS
UNICEF	United Nations Children's Fund
UNODC	United Nations Office on Drugs and Crime
VCT	voluntary counselling and testing
WHO	World Health Organization
WHO GHP	WHO Global Hepatitis Programme

GLOSSARY OF TERMS

Markers for HBV infection

HB surface antigen (HBsAg)	HBV envelope protein often produced in excess and detectable in the blood in acute and chronic HBV infection
HB core antigen (HBcAg)	HBV core protein. The core protein is coated with HBsAg and therefore not found free in serum
HB e antigen (HBeAg)	Viral protein found in the high replicative phase of HBV. HBeAg is usually a marker of high levels of replication with wild-type virus but is not essential for viral replication
HB surface antibody (anti-HBs)	Antibody to HBsAg. Develops in response to hepatitis B vaccination and during recovery from hepatitis B, denoting past infection and immunity
HB core antibody (anti-HBc)	Antibody to HBV core (capsid) protein. Anti-HBc antibodies are non neutralizing antibodies and are detected in both acute and chronic infection
anti-HBc IgM	Subclass of anti-HBc. Detected in recent HBV infection but can be detected by sensitive assays in chronic HBV infection
HBV e antibody (anti-HBe)	Antibody to HBeAg. Detected in persons with lower levels of HBV replication but also in HBeAg-negative disease (i.e. HBV that does not express HBeAg)
HBV DNA	HBV viral genomes that can be detected and quantified in serum by nucleic acid testing (NAT)

Markers for HCV infection

Anti-HCV antibody	Antibody to HCV, which can be detected in the blood usually within two or three months of HCV infection or exposure. The terms HCV antibody and anti-HCV antibody are equivalent, but in these guidelines, HCV antibody is used throughout.
HCV RNA	HCV viral genomes that can be detected and quantified in serum by nucleic acid testing (NAT).
HCV core antigen (HCVcAg)	Nucleocapsid peptide 22 [p22] of HCV, which is released into plasma during viral assembly and can be detected from early on and throughout the course of infection

Natural history of viral hepatitis

Chronic HBV infection	Persistence of HBsAg for at least six months. The persistence of HBsAg in two specimens six months apart is frequently used in clinical practice to confirm chronic hepatitis B infection.

Chronic HCV infection	The presence of viraemic HCV RNA or HCVcAg in association with positive serology for HCV antibody.
Viraemic infection	Hepatitis B or C infection associated with presence of virus in the blood (as measured by HBV DNA or HCV RNA), and often referred to as active, ongoing or current infection.
Occult HBV infection	HBsAg negative but HBV DNA positive, although at very low levels (invariably <200 IU/mL). Most are also anti-HBc positive.
Cirrhosis	An advanced stage of liver disease characterized by extensive hepatic fibrosis, nodularity of the liver, alteration of liver architecture and disrupted hepatic circulation.
Decompensated cirrhosis	Clinical features are portal hypertension (ascites, variceal haemorrhage and hepatic encephalopathy), coagulopathy, or liver insufficiency (jaundice). Other clinical features of advanced liver disease/cirrhosis may include: hepatomegaly, splenomegaly, pruritus, fatigue, arthralgia, palmar erythema, and oedema.
Hepatocellular carcinoma (HCC)	Primary cancer of the liver arising from the hepatocytes and may be a complication of chronic hepatitis B or C infection

Measures of treatment response

HCV sustained virological response (SVR)	Undetectable HCV RNA in the blood at defined time point after the end of treatment, usually at 12 or 24 weeks (SVR12 or 24)
HCV non-response	Detectable HCV RNA in the blood throughout treatment
HCV relapse	Undetectable HCV RNA during treatment and/or at end of treatment, but subsequent detectable HCV RNA following treatment cessation
HCV viral breakthrough	Undetectable HCV RNA during treatment followed by detectable HCV RNA despite continued treatment
HBV treatment failure	May be primary or secondary. Primary antiviral treatment failure may be defined as failure of an antiviral drug to reduce HBV DNA levels by $\geq 1 \times \log_{10}$ IU/mL within 3 months of initiating therapy. Secondary antiviral treatment failure may be defined as a rebound of HBV DNA levels of $\geq 1 \times \log_{10}$ IU/mL from the nadir in persons with an initial antiviral treatment effect ($\geq 1 \times \log_{10}$ IU/mL decrease in serum HBV DNA).

Diagnostic testing for hepatitis B and hepatitis C

Serological assays	Assays that detect the presence of either antigens or antibodies, typically in serum or plasma but also in capillary/venous whole blood and oral fluid. These include rapid diagnostic tests (RDTs), and laboratory-based immunoassays, e.g. enzyme immunoassays (EIAs), chemiluminescence immunoassays (CLIAs), and electro-chemiluminescence immunoassays (ECLs).

Rapid diagnostic test (RDT)	Immunoassays that detect antibodies or antigens and can give a result in less than 30 minutes. Most RDTs can be performed with capillary whole blood collected by finger-stick sampling.
Enzyme immunoassay (EIA)	Laboratory-based serological immunoassays that detect antibodies, antigens, or a combination of both
Nucleic acid testing (NAT)	A molecular technology, for example, polymerase chain reaction (PCR) or nucleic acid sequence-based amplification (NASBA) that can detect very small quantities of viral nucleic acid (RNA or DNA), either qualitatively or quantitatively.
Multiplex or multi-disease testing	Refers to testing using one specimen in the same test device (or reagent cartridge) that can detect other infections (e.g. HIV, syphilis, hepatitis C, hepatitis B)

Measures of test performance

Clinical/diagnostic sensitivity of a test	The ability of a test to correctly identify those with the infection or disease (i.e. true positives/true positives + false negatives)
Clinical/diagnostic specificity of a test	The ability of a test to correctly identify those without the infection or disease (i.e. true negatives/true negatives + false positives) Sensitivity and specificity are usually expressed as point estimates accompanied by confidence intervals.
Positive predictive value (PPV)	The probability that when a person's test result is positive, they truly have the infection/disease
Negative predictive value (NPV)	The probability that when a person's test result is negative, they truly do not have the infection/disease Predictive values are influenced by the prevalence of the disease in the population.
Analytical sensitivity/Limit of detection (LoD)	The lowest concentration of measurement that can be consistently detected in 95% of specimens tested under routine laboratory conditions. It defines the analytical sensitivity in contrast to the clinical or diagnostic sensitivity.

Testing terminology

Testing algorithm	The combination and sequence of specific assays used within hepatitis B and C testing strategies
Testing approach	In the context of these guidelines, the testing approach describes both "who to test" i.e. different populations and "where to test" i.e different settings. Testing approaches include general population testing, focused testing of high-risk groups, "birth-cohort" testing or of antenatal clinics. These can be delivered through either health-facility or community-based testing.

| Testing strategy | A general sequence of assays for a specific testing objective or approach, taking into consideration the presumed disease prevalence in the population being tested. A one-assay serological testing strategy involves a single serological assay. A two-assay serological testing strategy involves two different serological assays used sequentially. |

Testing approaches terminology

Key populations	Groups of people who due to specific high-risk behaviours, are at increased risk for HIV infection irrespective of the epidemic type or local context. This may also apply to HBV and/or HCV infection. Key populations often have legal and social issues related to their behaviours that increase their vulnerability to HIV, HBV and HCV infection. These guidelines refer to the following groups as key populations: men who have sex with men (MSM); people who inject drugs (PWID); people in prisons and other closed settings; sex workers; and transgender people.
Vulnerable populations	Groups of people who are particularly vulnerable to HBV/HCV infection in certain situations or contexts. These guidelines refer to the following groups as vulnerable populations: migrant and mobile workers, and indigenous populations.
General population testing	This approach refers to routine testing throughout the entire population without attempting to identify high-risk behaviours or characteristics. It means that all members of the population should have potential access to the testing programme.
"Birth cohort" testing	This approach means routine testing among easily identified age or demographic groups (i.e. specific "birth cohorts") known to have a high HCV prevalence due to past generalized exposures that have since been identified and removed.
Antenatal clinic testing	This approach means routine testing of pregnant women especially in settings where there is an intermediate or high seroprevalence, to identify women in need of antiviral treatment for their own health and additional interventions to reduce mother-to-child transmission (MTCT)
Community-based testing	Includes using outreach (mobile) approaches in general and key populations; home-based testing (or door-to-door outreach); testing in workplaces, places of worship, parks, bars and other venues; in schools and other educational establishments; as well as through campaigns
Facility-based testing	Includes testing in primary care clinics, inpatient wards and outpatient clinics, including specialist dedicated clinics such as HIV, STI and TB clinics, in district, provincial or regional hospitals and their laboratories, and in private clinical services.

Service delivery terminology

Integration	The co-location and sharing of services and resources across different disease areas. In the context of hepatitis B or C infection, this may include the provision of testing, prevention, care and treatment services alongside other health services, such as HIV, tuberculosis (TB), sexually transmitted infections (STI), antenatal clinic (ANC), contraceptive and other family planning services.
Decentralization	The process of delegating significant authority and resources to lower levels of the health system (provincial, regional, district, sub-district, primary health care and community
Task-shifting/ sharing	The rational redistribution of tasks from "higher-level" cadres of health-care providers to other cadres, such as trained lay providers
Lay provider	Any person who performs functions related to health-care delivery and has been trained to deliver services but has received no formal professional or paraprofessional certificate or tertiary education degree
Linkage to care	A process of actions and activities that support people testing for HBV/HCV to engage with prevention, treatment and care services as appropriate for their hepatitis B and C status.

EXECUTIVE SUMMARY

Background

Hepatitis B virus (HBV) and hepatitis C virus (HCV) infection are major causes of acute and chronic liver disease (e.g. cirrhosis and hepatocellular carcinoma) globally, and cause an estimated 1.4 million deaths annually. It is estimated that, at present, 248 million people are living with chronic HBV infection, and that 110 million persons are HCV-antibody positive, of which 80 million have active viraemic infection. The burden of chronic HBV and HCV remains disproportionately high in low- and middle-income countries (LMICs), particularly in Asia and Africa. Additionally, even in low-prevalence areas, certain populations have high levels of HCV and HBV infection, such as persons who inject drugs (PWID), men who have sex with men (MSM), people with HIV, as well as those belonging to certain indigenous communities.

The development of highly effective, well-tolerated oral direct acting antiviral (DAA) treatment regimens with high rates of cure after 8–12 weeks of treatment has revolutionized the treatment of chronic HCV infection, although the high prices of these new medicines remain a major barrier to access in many countries. Effective long-term antiviral treatment with tenofovir or entecavir is also available for people with chronic HBV infection. However, despite the high global burden of disease due to chronic HBV and HCV infection, and the advances and opportunities for treatment, most people infected with HBV and/or HCV remain unaware of their infection and therefore frequently present with advanced disease and may transmit infection to others. There are several key reasons for this low rate of hepatitis testing. These include the limited facilities or services for hepatitis testing, lack of effective testing policies or national guidelines, complex diagnostic algorithms, and poor laboratory capacity and quality assurance systems.

Testing and diagnosis of hepatitis B and C infection is the gateway for access to both prevention and treatment services, and is a crucial component of an effective response to the hepatitis epidemic. Early identification of persons with chronic HBV or HCV infection enables them to receive the necessary care and treatment to prevent or delay progression of liver disease. Testing also provides an opportunity to link people to interventions to reduce transmission, through counselling on risk behaviours and provision of prevention commodities (such as sterile needles and syringes) and hepatitis B vaccination.

About the guidelines

These are the first WHO guidelines on testing for chronic HBV and HCV infection and complement published guidance by WHO on the prevention, care and treatment of chronic hepatitis C and hepatitis B infection[1,2]. These guidelines outline the public health approach to strengthening and expanding current testing practices for HBV and HCV, and are intended for use across age groups and populations. The primary audience for these WHO guidelines are country programme managers and health-care providers, particularly in LMICs, responsible for planning and implementing hepatitis testing, prevention, care and treatment services.

The document is organized into three distinct sections:

Introduction – Part 1: Introductory chapters on epidemiology, natural history and in vitro diagnostic assays for hepatitis B and C virus infection.

Recommendations – Part 2: Nine chapters with summary of recommendations, evidence and rationale for recommendations covering:

- who to test for chronic hepatitis B and C infection (testing approaches)
- how to test serologically for chronic hepatitis B and C infection (testing strategies)
- how to confirm viraemic HBV and HCV infection to guide treatment decisions
- how to assess response to antiviral treatment for chronic hepatitis B and C infection
- use of dried blood spot (DBS) specimens for serology testing and virological testing for chronic hepatitis B and C infection
- interventions to promote uptake of testing and linkage to care.

Implementation – Part 3: Guidance to support implementation of these recommendations at country level which include a framework for country decision-making and planning in two key areas: how to organize hepatitis testing laboratory services (systems for selection and evaluation of assays and quality assurance systems) and how to plan the best strategic mix of testing approaches. There is also guidance on different service delivery models for testing; pre and post-test counselling; and tailored testing approaches in specific populations (e.g. PWID, prisoners, pregnant women, children and adolescents).

---

[1] Guidelines for the screening, care and treatment of persons with chronic hepatitis C infection. Updated version, April 2016. Geneva: World Health Organization; 2016.
[2] Guidelines for the prevention, care and treatment of persons with chronic hepatitis B infection. Geneva: World Health Organization; 2015.

FIG. 1. Organization of the guidelines along the continuum of care

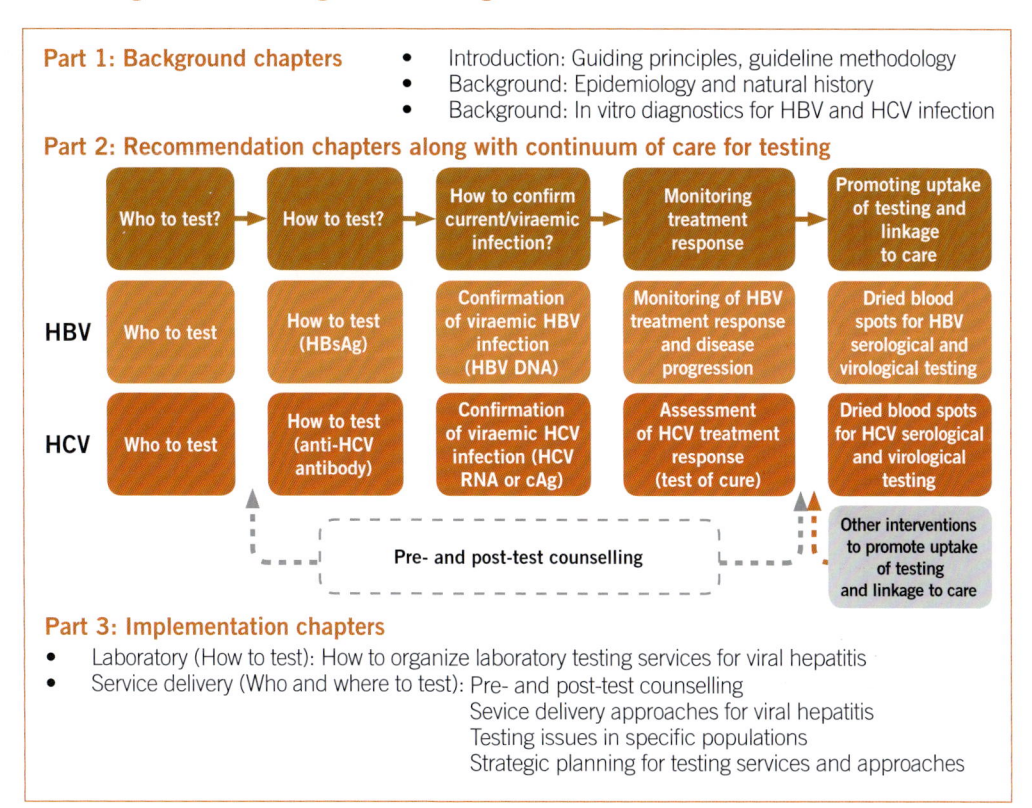

Part 1: Background chapters
- Introduction: Guiding principles, guideline methodology
- Background: Epidemiology and natural history
- Background: In vitro diagnostics for HBV and HCV infection

Part 2: Recommendation chapters along with continuum of care for testing

	Who to test?	How to test?	How to confirm current/viraemic infection?	Monitoring treatment response	Promoting uptake of testing and linkage to care
HBV	Who to test	How to test (HBsAg)	Confirmation of viraemic HBV infection (HBV DNA)	Monitoring of HBV treatment response and disease progression	Dried blood spots for HBV serological and virological testing
HCV	Who to test	How to test (anti-HCV antibody)	Confirmation of viraemic HCV infection (HCV RNA or cAg)	Assessment of HCV treatment response (test of cure)	Dried blood spots for HCV serological and virological testing

Pre- and post-test counselling

Other interventions to promote uptake of testing and linkage to care

Part 3: Implementation chapters
- Laboratory (How to test): How to organize laboratory testing services for viral hepatitis
- Service delivery (Who and where to test): Pre- and post-test counselling
  - Sevice delivery approaches for viral hepatitis
  - Testing issues in specific populations
  - Strategic planning for testing services and approaches

Summary of recommendations

Table 1 summarizes the recommendations on who to test (i.e. testing approaches); how to test (i.e. testing strategies), and interventions to promote uptake of testing and linkage to care. Figures 2 and 3 show summary algorithms for diagnosis, monitoring and management of chronic hepatitis B and C infection.

Who to test for HBV and HCV infection – testing approaches

The guidelines recommend offering focused testing to individuals from populations most affected by HBV or HCV infection (i.e. who are either part of a population with higher seroprevalence or who have a history of exposure to or high-risk behaviours for HBV or HCV infection). In settings with a ≥2% or ≥5% seroprevalence of hepatitis B surface antigen (HBsAg) or HCV antibody (anti-HCV) (based on existing published thresholds for intermediate or high seroprevalence, respectively), it is recommended that all adults have routine access to and be offered testing (i.e. a general population testing approach), or use "birth cohort" testing for specific age groups with higher anti-HCV seroprevalence. However, the threshold used by a country will depend on other country considerations and epidemiological context. Overall, these different testing approaches should make use of existing facility-based (such as antenatal clinics, HIV or TB services) or community- based testing opportunities and programmes.

How to test for HBV and HCV infection – serological assays and testing strategies

Overall, the guidelines recommend the use of a single quality-assured serological in vitro diagnostic test (i.e. either a laboratory-based immunoassay [enzyme immunoassay or chemiluminiscence immunoassay] or rapid diagnostic test [RDT]) to detect HBsAg and HCV antibody. RDTs used should meet minimum performance standards, and be delivered at the point of care to improve access and linkage to care and treatment.

Confirming viraemic infection and monitoring for treatment response

Following a reactive HCV antibody serological test result, a quantitative or qualitative RNA NAT is recommended as the preferred testing strategy to diagnose viraemic infection. Detection of core HCV antigen, where the assay has comparable clinical sensitivity to NAT technologies, may be considered as an alternative. The use of HBV DNA NAT following a reactive HBsAg serological test result, is recommended to help further guide who to treat or not treat if there is no evidence of cirrhosis, and to monitor for treatment response, based on existing recommendations from the 2015 WHO HBV management guidelines.

Use of dried blood spot sampling and other strategies to promote testing uptake and linkage to care

The use of capillary whole blood DBS specimens for both serological and NAT technologies for HBV and HCV infection may be considered to facilitate access to testing in certain settings where there are either no facilities or expertise to take venous blood specimens, in persons with poor venous access, or where quality-assured RDTs are not available or their use is not feasible. Programmes should consider only the use of assays that have been validated by their manufacturer for use with DBS specimens. Other recommended interventions to promote uptake of hepatitis testing and linkage to care include peer and lay health worker support in community- based settings, clinician reminders in facilities, and testing as part of integrated services within drug treatment and community-based harm reduction services.

The development of these guidelines was conducted in accordance with procedures established by the WHO Guidelines Review Committee. Clinical recommendations were formulated by a regionally representative and multidisciplinary Guidelines Development Group at a meeting held in September 2015. The GRADE (Grading of Recommendations Assessment, Development and Evaluation) approach was used to formulate and categorize strength of recommendations (strong or conditional), and was adapted for diagnostic tests. This includes an assessment of the quality of evidence (high, moderate, low or very low), consideration of overall balance of benefits and harms (at individual and population levels), patient/health worker values and preferences, resource use, cost–effectiveness and consideration of feasibility and effectiveness across a variety of resource-limited settings, including where access to laboratory infrastructure and specialized tests is limited. There was a very limited evidence base to guide recommendations on testing approaches (i.e. who to test and service delivery approaches) and an absence of evidence on patient-important outcomes in evaluation of performance of diagnostic tests and testing strategies. The process also identified key gaps in knowledge that will guide the future research agenda. Most of the evidence was based on published studies in adults from Asia, North America and Western Europe; there is a lack of data from sub-Saharan Africa, and in children.

Implementation of these recommendations pose practical challenges to policy-makers and implementers in LMICs, particularly in sub-Saharan Africa, where there is currently very limited access to diagnostic tests, antiviral therapies and appropriate laboratory infrastructure. These guidelines also provide the framework for country decision-making and planning for hepatitis laboratory testing programmes to ensure the quality and accuracy of hepatitis testing, as well as approaches to delivery of testing services, including opportunities to integrate hepatitis testing with existing services, where appropriate.

These guidelines and recommendations provide a major opportunity to improve identification and treatment of persons with chronic hepatitis B and C, and achieve the Global Hepatitis Health Sector Strategy (GHSS) on Viral Hepatitis [3] targets, including those on testing (i.e. identify 30% of persons living with HBV and HCV by 2020 and 90% by 2030). This in turn will improve clinical outcomes and save lives, as well as facilitate prevention, reducing hepatitis transmission and new infections.

---

[3] WHO Global health sector strategy on viral hepatitis 2016–2021. Geneva: World Health Organization; 2016.

SUMMARY ALGORITHMS

FIG.2. Summary algorithm for diagnosis, treatment and monitoring[1] of chronic HBV infection

1. SEROLOGICAL TESTING

HEPATITIS B SURFACE ANTIGEN (HBsAg)
Single RDT[2] or laboratory-based immunoassay[3]

- HBsAg + (reactive) Report positive → Compatible with HBV infection
- HBsAg − (non-reactive) Report negative → No serological evidence of HBV infection

2. ASSESSMENT FOR TREATMENT

ASSESSMENT OF STAGE OF LIVER DISEASE
(using clinical criteria[4] and/or non-invasive tests (NITs) for presence of cirrhosis, i.e. APRI score[5] >2 or based on TE[6])

HBV DNA NUCLEIC ACID TEST (NAT) (quantitative)
(to further guide who to treat and not treat, if no evidence of cirrhosis)

PRESENCE OF CIRRHOSIS

- **Yes** →
  - **ALL AGES** >30 years (in particular)
  - ALT[7,8] Persistently abnormal
  - HBV DNA >20 000 IU/mL
  - → **INITIATE ANTIVIRAL THERAPY[9] AND MONITOR**
    - Tenofovir or entecavir
    - Entecavir in children aged 2–11 years

- **No** →
  - ALT[7] Intermittently abnormal — HBV DNA 2000–20 000 IU/mL
  - ALT[7] Persistently normal — HBV DNA <2000 IU/mL
  - **AGE ≤30 years**: ALT[7] Persistently normal — HBV DNA <2000 IU/mL
  - → **DEFER TREATMENT AND MONITOR**

3. MONITORING

DETECTION OF HCC in persons with cirrhosis or HCC family history (every 6 months)
- Ultrasound and serum AFP

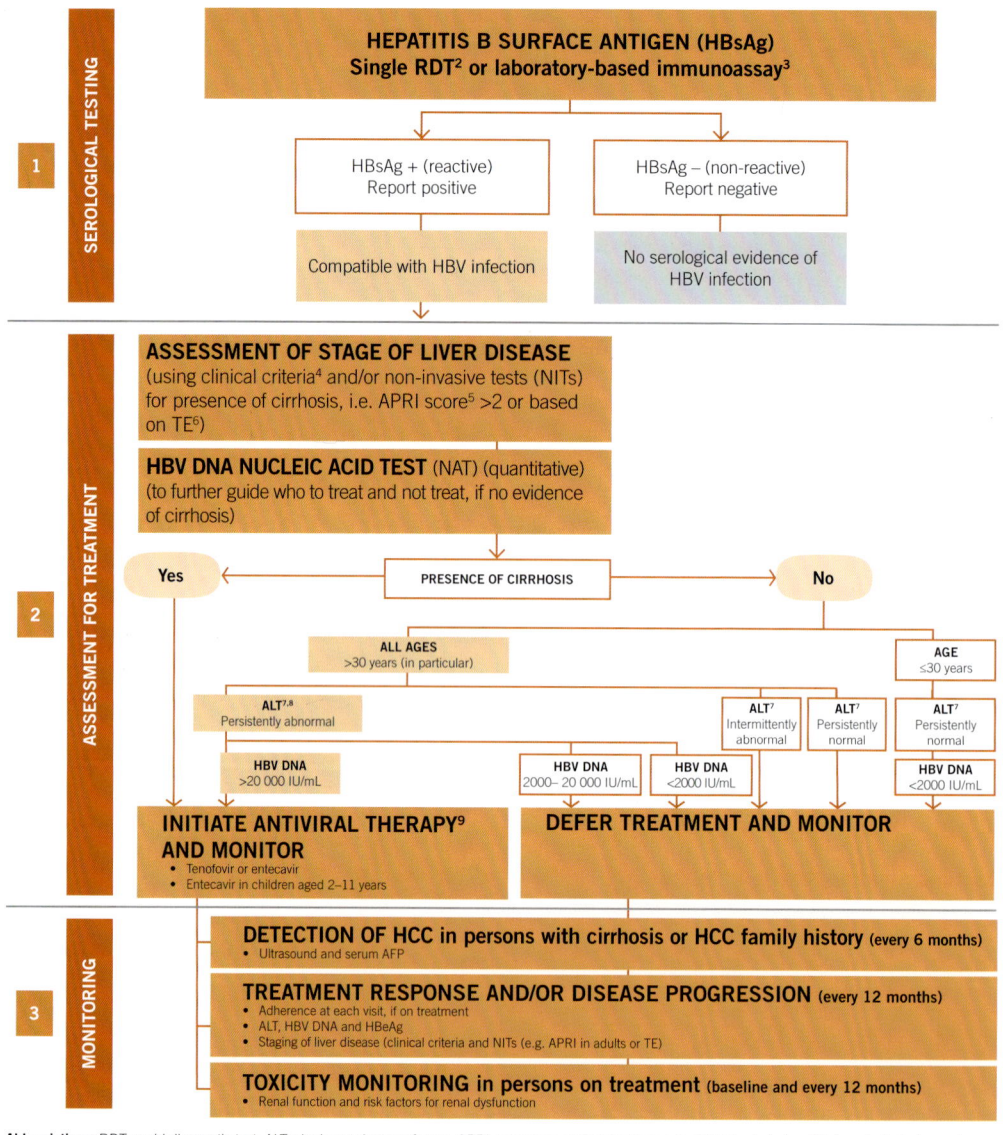

TREATMENT RESPONSE AND/OR DISEASE PROGRESSION (every 12 months)
- Adherence at each visit, if on treatment
- ALT, HBV DNA and HBeAg
- Staging of liver disease (clinical criteria and NITs (e.g. APRI in adults or TE)

TOXICITY MONITORING in persons on treatment (baseline and every 12 months)
- Renal function and risk factors for renal dysfunction

Abbreviations: RDT: rapid diagnostic test; ALT: alanine aminotransferase; APRI: aspartase aminotransferase-to-platelet ratio index; TE: transient elastography; HCC: hepatocellular carcinoma; AFP: apha fetoprotein

[1] Guidelines for the prevention, care and treatment of persons with chronic hepatitis B infection. Geneva: World Health Organization; 2015.
[2] In settings or populations with a low HBsAg seroprevalence <0.4%, confirmation of HBsAg positivity on the same immunoassay with a neutralization step or a second different RDT assay for detection of HBsAg may be considered.
[3] Laboratory-based Immunoassays include enzyme immunoassay (EIA), chemiluminescence immunoassay (CLIA), and electrochemoluminescence assay (ECL)
[4] Decompensated cirrhosis is defined by the development of portal hypertension (ascites, variceal haemorrhage and hepatic encephalopathy), coagulopathy, or liver insufficiency (jaundice). Other clinical features of advanced liver disease/cirrhosis may include: hepatomegaly, splenomegaly, pruritus, fatigue, arthralgia, palmar erythema, and oedema.
[5] Aspartate aminotransferase (AST)-to-platelet ratio index (APRI) is a simple index for estimating hepatic fibrosis based on a formula derived from AST and platelet concentrations.
The formula for calculating the APRI score is: APRI = (AST/AST ULN) x 100) /platelet count (10^9/L). Most recommend using 40 IU/L as the value for AST upper limit of normal (ULN).
An online calculator can be found at: http://www.hepatitisc.uw.edu/page/clinical-calculators/apri
[6] Transient elastography (Fibroscan): a technique to measure liver stiffness (as a surrogate for fibrosis)
[7] ALT levels fluctuate in persons with chronic hepatitis B and require longitudinal monitoring to determine the trend. Upper limits for normal ALT have been defined as below 30 U/L for men and 19 U/L for women, though local laboratory normal ranges should be applied. Persistently normal/abnormal may be defined as three ALT determinations below or above the upper limit of normal, made at unspecified intervals during a 6–12-month period or predefined intervals during a 12-month period.
[8] Where HBV DNA testing is not available, treatment may be considered based on persistently abnormal ALT levels, but other common causes of persistently raised ALT levels such as impaired glucose tolerance, dyslipidaemia and fatty liver should be excluded.
[9] Initiate antiviral therapy with tenofovir alone only after exclusion of HIV coinfection.

FIG.3. Summary algorithm for diagnosis, treatment and monitoring[1] of chronic HCV infection

1 SEROLOGICAL TESTING

ANTI-HCV ANTIBODY
Single RDT or laboratory-based immunoassay[2]

- Anti-HCV + (reactive) — Report positive
  - Compatible with current or past HCV infection
- Anti-HCV – (non-reactive) — Report negative
  - No serological evidence of HCV infection

2 CONFIRMATION OF VIRAEMIC INFECTION

HCV RNA NUCLEIC ACID TEST (NAT)
(qualitative or quantitative) or HCV core antigen (cAg)

- HCV RNA test or cAg + — Report detected (with viral load if available)
  - Compatible with viraemic HCV infection
- HCV RNA test or cAg – — Report not detected
  - No current viraemic HCV

3 TREATMENT ASSESSMENT

ASSESSMENT OF STAGE OF LIVER DISEASE (using clinical criteria[3] and non-invasive tests (NITs), i.e. APRI score[4] >2 or based on TE[5])

OTHER CONSIDERATIONS FOR TREATMENT (e.g. comorbidities, HCV genotyping, pregnancy and potential drug-drug interactions)

FACTORS TO BE CONSIDERED IN PRIORITIZING TREATMENT
1. **Increased risk of death** (e.g. advanced fibrosis and cirrhosis, post-liver transplantation)
2. **Risk of accelerated fibrosis** (e.g. HIV or HBV coinfection, metabolic syndrome, high level of alcohol use)
3. **Extrahepatic manifestations and evidence of end-organ damage** (e.g. debilitating fatigue, vasculitis and lymphoproliferative disorders)
4. **Significant psychosocial morbidity** (e.g. due to stigma, discrimination, fear of transmission to others)
5. **Maximizing reduction in incidence** (e.g. in PWID, MSM, prisoners, sex workers, women of childbearing age, health-care workers)

SELECT DIRECT-ACTING ANTIVIRAL (DAA) REGIMEN[1,6]
Daclatasvir/sofosbuvir or ledipasvir/sofosbuvir ± ribavirin for 12 or 24 weeks (depending on genotype and presence of cirrhosis)

4 MONITORING

ASSESSMENT OF CURE (sustained virological response (SVR) at 12 weeks (i.e. SVR12) after the end of treatment)
HCV RNA NAT (qualitative or quantitative)

DETECTION OF HCC in persons with cirrhosis (every 6 months)
Ultrasound and AFP

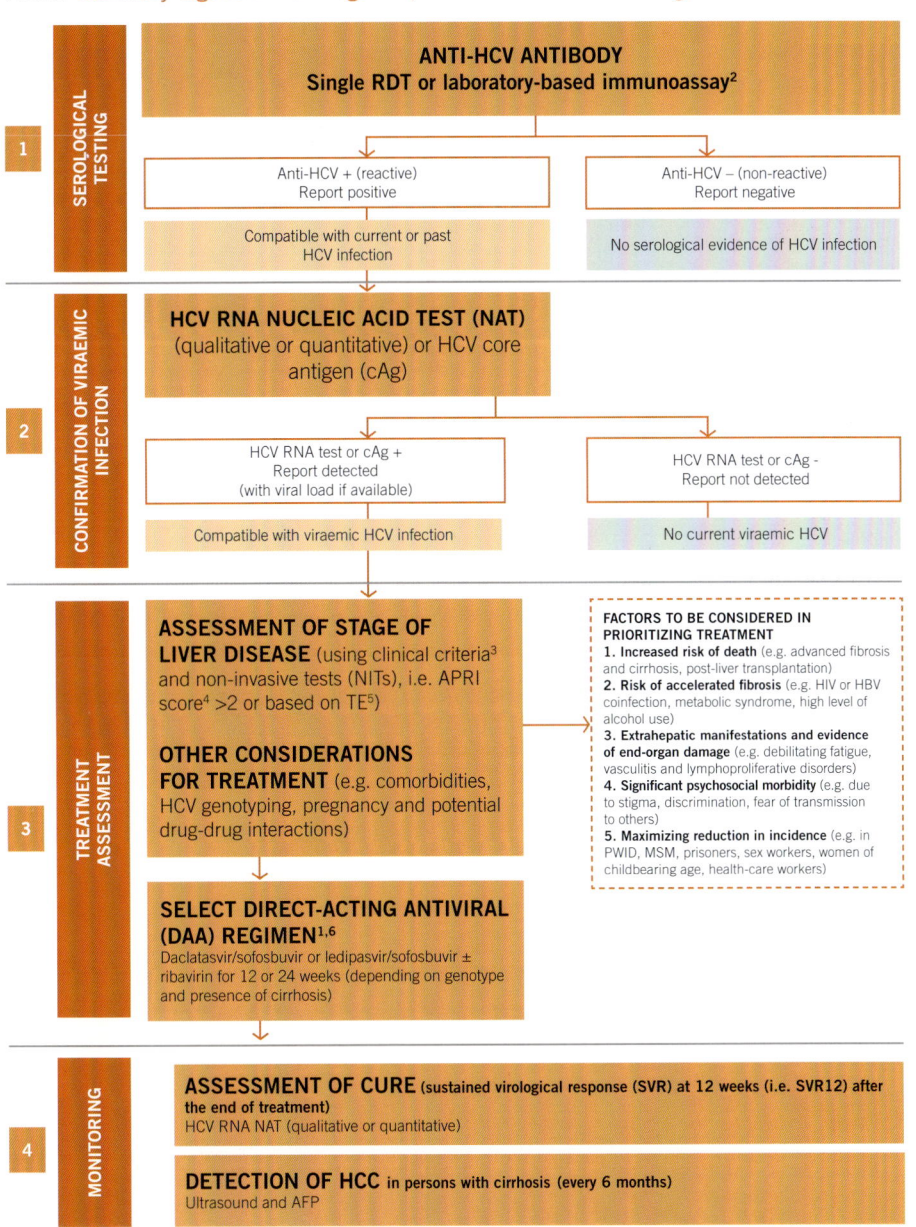

Abbreviations: RDT: rapid diagnostic test; APRI: aspartase aminotransferase-to-platelet ratio index, TE: transient elastography; PWID: people who inject drugs; MSM: men who have sex with men; HCC: hepatocellular carcinoma; AFP: alpha fetoprotein

[1] Guidelines for the screening, care and treatment of persons with chronic hepatitis C infection. Updated version, April 2016. Geneva: World Health Organization; 2016.
[2] Laboratory-based immunoassays include enzyme immunoassay (EIA), chemoluminescence immunoassay (CLIA), and electrochemoluminescence assay (ECL).
[3] Decompensated cirrhosis is defined by the development of portal hypertension (ascites, variceal haemorrhage and hepatic encephalopathy), coagulopathy, or liver insufficiency (jaundice). Other clinical features of advanced liver disease/cirrhosis may include: hepatomegaly, splenomegaly, pruritus, fatigue, arthralgia, palmar erythema, and oedema.
[4] Aspartate aminotransferase (AST)-to-platelet ratio index (APRI) is a simple index for estimating hepatic fibrosis based on a formula derived from AST and platelet concentrations. The formula for calculating the APRI score is: APRI = (AST/AST ULN) x 100) /platelet count (10^9/L). Most recommend using 40 IU/L as the value for AST upper limit of normal (ULN). An online calculator can be found at: http://www.hepatitisc.uw.edu/page/clinical-calculators/apri
[5] Transient elastography (Fibroscan) is a technique to measure liver stiffness (as a surrogate for fibrosis).
[6] Caution: there is a potential but uncertain risk of HBV reactivation during or after HCV clearance. Prior to starting DAA therapy, test for HBV infection (HBsAg, HBeAg, and HBV DNA) to assess indication for HBV treatment. Continue careful monitoring after completion of DAA therapy, including for HCC.

TABLE 1. SUMMARY OF RECOMMENDATIONS ON TESTING FOR CHRONIC HEPATITIS B AND C VIRUS INFECTION

WHO TO TEST FOR CHRONIC HBV INFECTION

Testing approach and population	Recommendations*
General population testing	1. In settings with a ≥2% or ≥5%[1] HBsAg seroprevalence in the general population, it is recommended that all adults have routine access to and be offered HBsAg serological testing with linkage to prevention, care and treatment services. General population testing approaches should make use of existing community- or health facility-based testing opportunities or programmes such as at antenatal clinics, HIV or TB clinics. *Conditional recommendation, low quality of evidence*
Routine testing in pregnant women	2. In settings with a ≥2% or ≥5%%[1] HBsAg seroprevalence in the general population, it is recommended that HBsAg serological testing be routinely offered to all pregnant women in antenatal clinics[2], with linkage to prevention, care and treatment services. Couples and partners in antenatal care settings should be offered HBV testing services. *Strong recommendation, low quality of evidence*
Focused testing in most affected populations	3. In all settings (and regardless of whether delivered through facility- or community-based testing), it is recommended that HBsAg serological testing and linkage to care and treatment services be offered to the following individuals: • **Adults and adolescents from populations most affected by HBV infection**[3] (i.e. who are either part of a population with high HBV seroprevalence or who have a history of exposure and/or high-risk behaviours for HBV infection); • **Adults, adolescents and children with a clinical suspicion of chronic viral hepatitis**[4] (i.e. symptoms, signs, laboratory markers); • **Sexual partners, children and other family members, and close household contacts** of those with HBV infection[5]; • **Health-care workers:** in all settings, it is recommended that HBsAg serological testing be offered and hepatitis B vaccination given to all health-care workers who have not been vaccinated previously (*adapted from existing guidance on hepatitis B vaccination*[6]) *Strong recommendation, low quality of evidence*
Blood donors *Adapted from existing 2010 WHO guidance (Screening donated blood for transfusion transmissible infections*[7]*)*	4. In all settings, screening of blood donors should be mandatory with linkage to care, counselling and treatment for those who test positive.

Abbreviations: HBsAg: hepatitis B surface antigen; PWID: people who inject drugs; MSM: men who have sex with men
*The GRADE system (Grading of Recommendations, Assessment, Development and Evaluation) was used to categorize the strength of recommendations as strong or conditional (based on consideration of the quality of evidence, balance of benefits and harms, acceptability, resource use and programmatic feasibility) and the quality of evidence as high, moderate, low or very low.

[1] A threshold of ≥2% or ≥5% seroprevalence was based on several published thresholds of intermediate or high seroprevalence. The threshold used will depend on other country considerations and epidemiological context.
[2] Many countries have chosen to adopt routine testing in all pregnant women, regardless of seroprevalence in the general population, and particularly where seroprevalence ≥2%. A full vaccination schedule including birth dose should be completed in all infants, in accordance with the WHO position paper on hepatitis B vaccines 2009.[6]
[3] Includes those who are either part of a population with higher seroprevalence (e.g. some mobile/migrant populations from high/intermediate endemic countries, and certain indigenous populations) or who have a history of exposure or high-risk behaviours for HBV infection (e.g. PWID, people in prisons and other closed settings, MSM and sex workers, HIV-infected persons, partners, family members and children of HBV-infected persons).
[4] Features that may indicate underlying chronic HBV infection include clinical evidence of existing liver disease, such as cirrhosis or hepatocellular carcinoma (HCC), or where there is unexplained liver disease, including abnormal liver function tests or liver ultrasound.
[5] In all settings, it is recommended that HBsAg serological testing with hepatitis B vaccination of those who are HBsAg negative and not previously vaccinated be offered to all children with parents or siblings diagnosed with HBV infection or with clinical suspicion of hepatitis, through community- or facility-based testing.
[6] WHO position paper. Hepatitis B vaccines. Weekly Epidemiological Record. 2009;4 (84):405–20.
[7] Screening donated blood for transfusion transmissible infections. Geneva: World Health Organization; 2010.

WHO TO TEST FOR CHRONIC HCV INFECTION	
Testing approach and population	**Recommendations***
Focused testing in most affected populations	1. In all settings (and regardless of whether delivered through facility- or community-based testing), it is recommended that serological testing for HCV antibody (anti-HCV)[1] be offered with linkage to prevention, care and treatment services to the following individuals: • **Adults and adolescents from populations most affected by HCV infection**[2] (i.e. who are either part of a population with high HCV seroprevalence or who have a history of exposure and/or high-risk behaviours for HCV infection); • **Adults, adolescents and children with a clinical suspicion of chronic viral hepatitis**[3] (i.e. symptoms, signs, laboratory markers). *Strong recommendation, low quality of evidence* Note: Periodic re-testing using HCV NAT should be considered for those with ongoing risk of acquisition or reinfection.
General population testing	2. In settings with a ≥2% or ≥5%[4] HCV antibody seroprevalence in the general population, it is recommended that all adults have access to and be offered HCV serological testing with linkage to prevention, care and treatment services. General population testing approaches should make use of existing community- or facility-based testing opportunities or programmes such as HIV or TB clinics, drug treatment services and antenatal clinics[5]. *Conditional recommendation, low quality of evidence*
Birth cohort testing	3. This approach may be applied to specific identified birth cohorts of older persons at higher risk of infection[6] and morbidity within populations that have an overall lower general prevalence. *Conditional recommendation, low quality of evidence*

Abbreviations: NAT: nucleic acid test; anti-HCV: HCV antibody; PWID: people who inject drugs; MSM: men who have sex with men
*The GRADE system (Grading of Recommendations, Assessment, Development and Evaluation) was used to categorize the strength of recommendations as strong or conditional (based on consideration of the quality of evidence, balance of benefits and harms, acceptability, resource use and programmatic feasibility) and the quality of evidence as high, moderate, low or very low.

[1] This may include fourth-generation combined antibody/antigen assays
[2] Includes those who are either part of a population with higher seroprevalence (e.g. some mobile/migrant populations from high/intermediate endemic countries, and certain indigenous populations) or who have a history of exposure or high-risk behaviours for HCV infection (e.g. PWID, people in prisons and other closed settings, MSM and sex workers, and HIV-infected persons, children of mothers with chronic HCV infection especially if HIV-coinfected).
[3] Features that may indicate underlying chronic HCV infection include clinical evidence of existing liver disease, such as cirrhosis or hepatocellular carcinoma (HCC), or where there is unexplained liver disease, including abnormal liver function tests or liver ultrasound.
[4] A threshold of ≥2% or ≥5% seroprevalence was based on several published thresholds of intermediate and high seroprevalence. The threshold used will depend on other country considerations and epidemiological context.
[5] Routine testing of pregnant women for HCV infection is currently not recommended.
[6] Because of historical exposure to unscreened or inadequately screened blood products and/or poor injection safety.

HOW TO TEST FOR CHRONIC HBV INFECTION AND MONITOR TREATMENT RESPONSE

Topic	Recommendations*

Which serological assays to use	• For the diagnosis of chronic HBV infection in adults, adolescents and children (>12 months of age[1]), a serological assay (in either RDT or laboratory-based immunoassay format[2]) that meets minimum quality, safety and performance standards[3] (*with regard to both analytical and clinical sensitivity and specificity*) is recommended to detect hepatitis B surface antigen (HBsAg).
	   - In settings where existing laboratory testing is already available and accessible, laboratory-based immunoassays are recommended as the preferred assay format.
	   - In settings where there is limited access to laboratory testing and/or in populations where access to rapid testing would facilitate linkage to care and treatment, use of RDTs is recommended to improve access.
	Strong recommendation, low/moderate quality of evidence

Serological testing strategies	• In settings or populations with an HBsAg seroprevalence of ≥0.4%[4], a single serological assay for detection of HBsAg is recommended, prior to further evaluation for HBV DNA and staging of liver disease. • In settings or populations with a low HBsAg seroprevalence of <0.4%[4], confirmation of HBsAg positivity on the same immunoassay with a neutralization step or a second different RDT assay for detection of HBsAg may be considered[5]. *Conditional recommendation, low quality of evidence*
Detection of HBV DNA – assessment for treatment *Adapted from existing guidance (WHO HBV 2015 guidelines[6])*	• Directly following a positive HBsAg serological test, the use of quantitative or qualitative nucleic acid testing (NAT) for detection of HBV DNA is recommended as the preferred strategy and to guide who to treat or not treat. *Strong recommendation, moderate/low quality of evidence*

Monitoring for HBV treatment response and disease progression
Existing guidance (WHO HBV 2015 guidelines[6])
	• **It is recommended that the following be monitored at least annually:**
	   - ALT levels (and AST for APRI), HBsAg[7], HBeAg[8], and HBV DNA levels (where HBV DNA testing is available)
	   - Non-invasive tests (APRI score or transient elastography) to assess for presence of cirrhosis in those without cirrhosis at baseline;
	   - If on treatment, adherence should be monitored regularly and at each visit.
	Strong recommendation, moderate quality of evidence
	
	More frequent monitoring is recommended:
	• **In persons on treatment or following treatment discontinuation:** more frequent on-treatment monitoring (at least every 3 months for the first year) is indicated in: persons with more advanced disease (compensated or decompensated cirrhosis[9]); during the first year of treatment to assess treatment response and adherence; where treatment adherence is a concern; in HIV-coinfected persons; and in persons after discontinuation of treatment. *Conditional recommendation, very low quality of evidence*
	• **In persons who do not yet meet the criteria for antiviral therapy:** i.e. persons who have intermittently abnormal ALT levels or HBV DNA levels that fluctuate between 2000 IU/mL and 20 000 IU/mL (where HBV DNA testing is available) and in HIV-coinfected persons[7]. *Conditional recommendation, low quality of evidence*

Abbreviations: ALT: alanine aminotransferase; AST: aspartate aminotransferase; APRI: aspartate-to-platelet ratio index; HBeAg: HBV e antigen; HBsAg: HBV surface antigen; NAT: nucleic acid test; RDT: rapid diagnostic test

[1] A full vaccination schedule including birth dose should be completed in all infants in accordance with the WHO position paper on Hepatitis B vaccines, 2009. Testing of exposed infants is problematic within the first six months of life as HBsAg and hepatitis B DNA may be inconsistently detectable in infected infants. Exposed infants should be tested for HBsAg between 6 and 12 months of age to screen for evidence of hepatitis B infection. In all age groups, acute HBV infection can be confirmed by the presence of HBsAg and IgM anti-HBc. CHB is diagnosed if there is persistence of HBsAg for six months or more.
[2] Laboratory-based immunoassays include enzyme immunoassay (EIA), chemoluminescence immunoassay (CLIA), and electrochemoluminescence assay (ECL).
[3] Assays should meet minimum acceptance criteria of either WHO prequalification of in vitro diagnostics (IVDs) or a stringent regulatory review for IVDs. All IVDs should be used in accordance with manufacturers' instructions for use and where possible at testing sites enrolled in a national or international external quality assessment scheme.
[4] Based on results of predictive modelling of positive predictive values according to different thresholds of seroprevalence in populations to be tested, and assay diagnostic performance.
[5] A repeat HBsAg assay after 6 months is also a common approach used to confirm chronicity of HBV infection.
[6] For further details, *see* Chapter 5: Who to treat and who not to treat. Guidelines for the prevention, care and treatment of persons with chronic hepatitis B infection: World Health Organization; 2015.
[7] In persons on treatment, monitor for HBsAg loss (although this occurs rarely), and for seroreversion to HBsAg positivity after discontinuation of treatment.
[8] Monitoring of HBeAg/anti-HBe mainly applies to those who are initially HBeAg positive. However, those who have already achieved HBeAg seroconversion and are HBeAg negative and anti-HBe positive may serorevert.
[9] Decompensated cirrhosis is defined by the development of portal hypertension (ascites, variceal haemorrhage and hepatic encephalopathy), coagulopathy, or liver insufficiency (jaundice). Other clinical features of advanced liver disease/cirrhosis may include: hepatomegaly, splenomegaly, pruritus, fatigue, arthralgia, palmar erythema and oedema.

HOW TO TEST FOR CHRONIC HCV INFECTION AND MONITOR TREATMENT RESPONSE	
Topic	**Recommendations***
Which serological assays to use	• To test for serological evidence of past or present infection in adults, adolescents and children (>18 months of age[1]), an HCV serological assay (antibody or antibody/antigen) using either RDT or laboratory-based immunoassay formats[2] that meet minimum safety, quality and performance standards[3] (*with regard to both analytical and clinical sensitivity and specificity*) is recommended. – In settings where there is limited access to laboratory infrastructure and testing, and/or in populations where access to rapid testing would facilitate linkage to care and treatment, RDTs are recommended. *Strong recommendation, low/moderate quality of evidence*
Serological testing strategies	In adults and children older than 18 months[1], a single serological assay for initial detection of serological evidence of past or present infection is recommended prior to supplementary nucleic acid testing (NAT) for evidence of viraemic infection. *Conditional recommendation, low quality of evidence*
Detection of viraemic infection	• Directly following a reactive HCV antibody serological test result, the use of quantitative or qualitative NAT for detection of HCV RNA is recommended as the preferred strategy to diagnose viraemic infection. *Strong recommendation, moderate/low quality of evidence* • An assay to detect HCV core (p22) antigen, which has comparable clinical sensitivity to NAT, is an alternative to NAT to diagnose viraemic infection[4]. *Conditional recommendation, moderate quality of evidence*
Assessment of HCV treatment response	• Nucleic acid testing for qualitative or quantitative detection of HCV RNA should be used as test of cure at 12 or 24 weeks (i.e. sustained virological response (SVR12 or SVR24)) after completion of antiviral treatment. *Conditional recommendation, moderate/low quality of evidence*

Abbreviations: DBS: dried blood spot; IVD: in vitro diagnostics; NAT: nucleic acid test; RDT: rapid diagnostic test
*The GRADE system (Grading of Recommendations, Assessment, Development and Evaluation) was used to categorize the strength of recommendations as strong or conditional (based on consideration of the quality of evidence, balance of benefits and harms, acceptability, resource use and programmatic feasibility) and the quality of evidence as high, moderate, low or very low.

[1] HCV infection can be confirmed in children under 18 months only by virological assays to detect HCV RNA, because transplacental maternal antibodies remain in the child's bloodstream up until 18 months of age, making test results from serology assays ambiguous.
[2] Laboratory-based immunoassays include enzyme immunoassay (EIA), chemoluminescence immunoassay (CLIA), and electrochemoluminescence assay (ECL).
[3] Assays should meet minimum acceptance criteria of either WHO prequalification of IVDs or a stringent regulatory review for IVDs. All IVDs should be used in accordance with manufacturers' instructions, and where possible at testing sites enrolled in a national or international external quality assessment scheme.
[4] A lower level of analytical sensitivity can be considered, if an assay is able to improve access (i.e. an assay that can be used at the point of care or suitable for dried blood spot [DBS] specimens) and/or affordability. An assay with a limit of detection of 3000 IU/mL or lower would be acceptable and would identify 95% of those with viraemic infection, based on available data.

INTERVENTIONS TO PROMOTE UPTAKE OF HEPATITIS TESTING AND LINKAGE TO CARE

USE OF DRIED BLOOD SPOT (DBS) SPECIMENS FOR SEROLOGY AND NUCLEIC ACID TESTING

Topic	Recommendations*
Serological testing	• The use of DBS specimens for HBsAg and HCV antibody serology testing[1] may be considered in settings where: - there are no facilities or expertise to take venous whole blood specimens; **or** - RDTs are not available or their use is not feasible; **or** - there are persons with poor venous access (e.g. in drug treatment programmes, prisons). *Conditional recommendation, moderate (HBV)/low (HCV) quality of evidence*
Detection of viraemia (nucleic acid testing)	• The use of DBS specimens to test for HBV DNA and HCV RNA for diagnosis of HBV and HCV viraemia[1], respectively, may be considered in settings where: - there is a lack of access to sites or nearby laboratory facilities for NAT, or provision for timely delivery of specimens to a laboratory; or - there are persons with poor venous access (e.g. in drug treatment programmes, prisons). *Conditional recommendation, low (HBV)/moderate (HCV) quality of evidence*

OTHER INTERVENTIONS TO IMPROVE UPTAKE OF TESTING AND LINKAGE TO CARE

Topic	Recommendations*
Uptake of testing and linkage to care	• All facility- and community-based hepatitis testing services should adopt and implement strategies to enhance uptake of testing and linkage to care. *Strong recommendation, moderate quality of evidence* • The following evidence-based interventions should be considered to promote uptake of hepatitis testing and linkage to care and treatment initiation: *(Conditional recommendations)* - **Peer and lay health worker support in community-based settings** *(moderate quality of evidence).* - **Clinician reminders** to prompt provider-initiated, facility-based HBV and HCV testing in settings that have electronic records or analogous reminder systems *(very low quality of evidence).* - **Provision of hepatitis testing as part of integrated services** within mental health/substance use services *(very low quality of evidence).*

*The GRADE system (Grading of Recommendations, Assessment, Development and Evaluation) was used to categorize the strength of recommendations as strong or conditional (based on consideration of the quality of evidence, balance of benefits and harms, acceptability, resource use and programmatic feasibility) and the quality of evidence as high, moderate, low or very low.

[1] Well-functioning laboratory specimens referral network and system for return of results should be in place to maximize the impact of DBS specimens. There are currently few assays where the manufacturer's instructions state that DBS specimens are validated for use. Therefore, currently use of DBS specimens would be considered "off-label".

PART 1: BACKGROUND

- Introductory chapters on objectives, scope and methodology of the guidelines
- Background to epidemiology, natural history, and serological and other markers of hepatitis B and C infection
- Background to diagnostics used to test for hepatitis B and C infection

1. INTRODUCTION

1.1. Current challenges in viral hepatitis testing

Globally, hepatitis B virus (HBV) and hepatitis C virus (HCV) infection are major causes of acute and chronic liver disease (e.g. cirrhosis and hepatocellular carcinoma [HCC]), resulting in an estimated 1.4 million deaths annually *(1)*. It is estimated that 248 million people are living with chronic HBV infection (CHB) *(2)*, and that 110 million persons are HCV-antibody positive and 80 million have chronic viraemic HCV infection *(3)*. Worldwide, it is estimated that a similar proportion of the total liver cancer mortality can be attributed to HCV (34 500) and HBV (30 000), with a smaller fraction due to alcohol *(1)*. The burden of HBV and HCV remains disproportionately high in low- and middle-income countries (LMICs). Approximately 60% of the world's population live in areas where HBV infection is highly endemic, particularly Asia and Africa. Additionally, even in low-prevalence areas, certain subpopulations have high levels of HCV and HBV infection, such as men who have sex with men (MSM), persons who inject drugs (PWID), people with HIV, as well as indigenous communities and migrants. The development of highly effective, well-tolerated, oral direct-acting antiviral (DAA) treatment regimens with high rates of cure has revolutionized the treatment of chronic HCV infection *(4)*, although the high prices of the new medicines remain a major barrier to access in many countries *(5)*. For people with chronic HBV infection, effective long-term suppressive treatment with tenofovir or entecavir is available *(6)*.

Despite the high global burden of disease due to chronic hepatitis B and C infection, and the advances and opportunities for treatment, most people infected with HBV and/or HCV remain unaware of their infection and therefore frequently present with advanced disease. The extent of this hidden burden is poorly documented, and largely based on limited data from higher-income settings *(7–10)*. However, in low-income settings, it is estimated that less than 5% are aware of their diagnosis. This contrasts with the considerable recent progress in HIV testing coverage, whereby now more than half of all people living with HIV globally are aware of their status *(11)*. Early identification of persons with chronic HBV or HCV infection would enable infected persons to receive the necessary care and treatment to prevent or delay the onset of liver disease and, in addition, prevent transmission by HBV vaccination of non-immune household contacts and sex partners.

There are several key reasons for this current low rate of hepatitis testing in LMICs. These include the limited facilities or services for hepatitis testing, lack of effective testing policies or national standards due to weak or non-existent hepatitis surveillance programmes to inform regional epidemiology and testing policies, costly and complex diagnostic assays and algorithms, poor laboratory capacity and infrastructure, and use of poor-quality test kits and reagents. In addition, in LMICs, HBV and HCV treatment remains unaffordable for those most in need, even if they have been diagnosed.

1.2. Goals of viral hepatitis testing

Testing and diagnosis of HBV and HCV infection is the gateway for access to both prevention as well as care and treatment services (Fig. 1.1), and is a crucial component of an effective response to the hepatitis epidemic.

The primary goals of testing are

1. to identify and link infected individuals, their partners and families to appropriate care and treatment services, and reduce hepatitis-related mortality by providing treatment to those in need through the use of direct-acting curative antiviral therapy for chronic hepatitis C and lifelong antiviral therapy for chronic hepatitis B infection;

2. to provide a link to preventive interventions to reduce transmission. For hepatitis, this includes provision of hepatitis B vaccination, and implementing individual- or facility-level prevention measures to reduce further transmission;

3. to monitor response to antiviral treatment.

Testing is also undertaken for other reasons that are not within the scope of these guidelines. These include: surveillance for both acute hepatitis (to detect outbreaks, monitor trends in incidence and identify risk factors for new incident infections) and chronic hepatitis (to estimate the prevalence of chronic infection and monitor trends in sentinel groups) *(12)*; and screening by blood transfusion services for hepatitis B and hepatitis C infection to exclude blood donations at risk of transmitting infections from donors to recipients.

FIG. 1.1. Cascade of viral hepatitis prevention, diagnosis, care and treatment

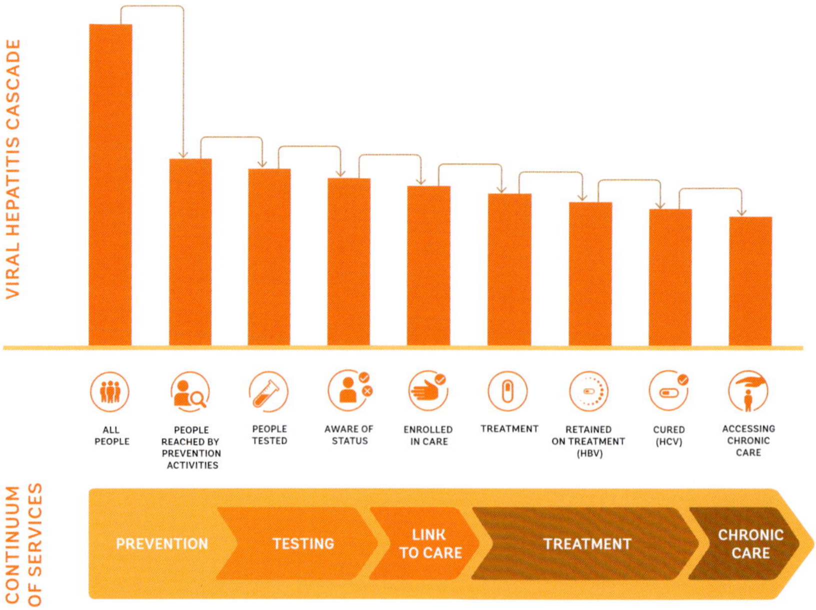

VIRAL HEPATITIS CASCADE

ALL PEOPLE | PEOPLE REACHED BY PREVENTION ACTIVITIES | PEOPLE TESTED | AWARE OF STATUS | ENROLLED IN CARE | TREATMENT | RETAINED ON TREATMENT (HBV) | CURED (HCV) | ACCESSING CHRONIC CARE

CONTINUUM OF SERVICES: PREVENTION → TESTING → LINK TO CARE → TREATMENT → CHRONIC CARE

Source: Global health sector strategy on viral hepatitis 2016–2021. Geneva, World Health Organization; 2016 *(16)*.

1.3. Why are testing guidelines needed?

In 2010 and 2014, World Health Assembly resolutions WHA63.18 *(13)* and WHA67 *(14)* recognized viral hepatitis as a global public health problem. It directed WHO to develop and implement both a comprehensive strategy to address viral hepatitis, as well as provide clear guidance to Member States on the diagnosis and management of HBV and HCV infection. Recent WHO guidelines on treatment for HCV *(5)* and HBV *(6)* did not include comprehensive guidance on who to test and how to test for diagnosis.

The Global Health Sector Strategy on Viral Hepatitis 2016–2021 *(16)* is the first global strategy on viral hepatitis, and covers the first six years of the Agenda for Sustainable Development. The Strategy outlines a set of global targets (*see Web annex 1*), including targets on diagnosis of chronic hepatitis B and hepatis C infection, and describes a set of priority actions for countries to achieve these hepatitis targets The Strategy is designed to contribute to the attainment of the 2030 Agenda for Sustainable Development and, specifically, to health-related Goal 3 (target 3.3). "By 2030, end the epidemics of AIDS, tuberculosis, malaria and neglected tropical diseases and combat hepatitis, water-borne diseases and other communicable diseases."

1.4. Goals and objectives of the guidelines

The overall objective of these guidelines is to provide the first WHO evidence-based guidance on testing for hepatitis B and C virus infection in adults, adolescents and children living, particularly in LMICs, where the burden of disease is highest and where access to treatment is becoming more readily available as treatment costs continue to decline. The guidelines are expected to provide the basis and rationale for the development of national guidelines for hepatitis testing, particularly in resource-limited settings, according to the local epidemiology of hepatitis B and C infection, health-care delivery system of the country, available resources and other determinants, with the overall aim of reducing the global burden of HBV and HCV infection.

The specific objectives of the guidelines are

- to provide recommendations in the area of who to screen for hepatitis B and hepatitis C infection, and which testing strategies and algorithms to use;

- to provide evidence summaries, Grading of Recommendations Assessment, Development and Evaluation (GRADE) reviews, evaluation of the overall balance of benefits and harms, feasibility, costs and acceptability of the proposed recommendations;

- to provide implementation guidance to support operationalization of the recommendations at country level, which includes a systematic approach to the selection and evaluation of assays, quality systems for all aspects of hepatitis testing, and a framework for planning the best mix of testing approaches;

- to identify research gaps.

1.5. Scope of the guidelines

The overall scope of these testing guidelines is the diagnosis, counselling and linkage to care of persons with chronic hepatitis B and hepatitis C infection. They are primarily aimed at resource-limited settings where hepatitis testing programmes are not yet well developed or where quality systems are lacking. The guidelines include the following components:

- testing approaches – who to test for chronic hepatitis B and C infection

- testing strategy – how to test for chronic hepatitis B and C infection

- interventions to promote uptake of hepatitis testing and linkage to care

- implementation issues with regard to product selection and procurement, validation of test kits, and quality assurance (QA).

Certain key topics were not included in the scope of work for these guidelines and are either addressed more fully in other WHO documents or guidelines, or will be included in future updates. These include: diagnosis and management of acute hepatitis B *(6)* and C infection *(5)*; surveillance of acute and chronic hepatitis B and hepatitis C *(12)*; treatment and side-effect monitoring of drugs for chronic hepatitis B and C *(5, 6, 15)*; diagnosis and management of hepatitis A *(17)*, hepatitis E *(18)* and hepatitis delta virus *(19)*; use of HCV RNA or core antigen as a single test for the diagnosis of HCV infection; and recommendations and testing strategies for screening of donated blood *(20)*.

1.6. Target audience

These guidelines are primarily targeted at national hepatitis programme managers and other policy-makers in ministries of health, particularly in LMICs, who are responsible for the development of national hepatitis testing and treatment plans, policy and guidelines. These guidelines will also be useful for laboratory managers in ministries of health, reference laboratories and key hospital laboratories, who are responsible for validation of assays, development of national testing algorithms, and national procurement of assays and quality control (QC). Finally, the guidelines will serve as a reference for health-care providers who offer and implement hepatitis testing and care for persons with hepatitis B and hepatitis C infection, including those from community-based programmes.

1.7. Related WHO materials and guidelines

These guidelines on testing for chronic hepatitis B and hepatitis C infection are intended to complement several existing WHO guidelines. These include the following:

Guidelines for the prevention, care and treatment of persons with chronic hepatitis B infection (http://apps.who.int/iris/bitstream/10665/154590/1/9789241549059_eng.pdf?ua=1&ua=1) *(6)* and **for chronic hepatitis C infection** (http://apps.who.int/iris/bitstream/10665/205035/1/9789241549615_eng.pdf) *(5)*. These provide recommendations along the continuum of care, from diagnosis, initial assessment of stage of liver disease, initiation of treatment and monitoring. A summary of recommendations is provided in *Web annexes 2* and *3,* respectively.

• **Consolidated guidelines on HIV testing services** (http://apps.who.int/iris/bitstream/10665/251655/1/9789241549868-eng.pdf?ua=1) *(11)* and **HIV self-testing supplement** (http://apps.who.int/iris/bitstream/10665/251655/1/9789241549868-eng.pdf?ua=1) *(21)*.

• **Technical considerations and case definitions to improve surveillance for viral hepatitis (**http://apps.who.int/iris/bitstream/10665/204501/1/9789241549547_

eng.pdf) *(12)* and **Monitoring and evaluation for viral hepatitis B and C: recommended indicators and framework: technical report** (http://apps.who.int/iris/bitstream/10665/204790/1/9789241510288_eng.pdf?ua=1) *(22)*.

- **Consolidated guidelines on the use of antiretroviral drugs for treating and preventing HIV infection** (http://apps.who.int/iris/bitstream/10665/208825/1/9789241549684_eng.pdf?ua=1) *(23)*.

- **Hepatitis B control through immunization: a reference guide** on prevention of perinatal and early childhood HBV infection through infant hepatitis B vaccination *(24)* (http://www.who.int/immunization/sage/meetings/2015/october/8_WPRO_Hepatitis_B_Prevention_Through_Immunization_Regional_Reference_Guide.pdf); as well as catch-up vaccinations in key affected populations (http://apps.who.int/iris/bitstream/10665/128048/1/9789241507431_eng.pdf?ua=1&ua=1 ns) *(25)*, such as PWID, MSM *(26)* and sex workers *(27)* (http://apps.who.int/iris/bitstream/10665/44619/1/9789241501750_eng.pdf?ua=1); (https://www.unfpa.org/sites/default/files/pub-pdf/9789241504744_eng.pdf).

- **Consolidated guidelines on HIV prevention, diagnosis, treatment and care for key populations** *(25)* and **Guidance on prevention of viral hepatitis B and C among people who inject drugs** (http://apps.who.int/iris/bitstream/10665/75357/1/9789241504041_eng.pdf?ua=1) *(28)*.

- **Guidance on prevention of hepatitis infection in health-care settings** *(28–30)* includes recommendations on hand hygiene, including surgical hand preparation, handwashing and use of gloves; safe handling and disposal of sharps and waste; safe cleaning of equipment; testing of donated blood and blood products; improved access to safe blood and blood products; and training of health personnel. There are also new WHO recommendations published in 2015 on the use of auto-disable syringes in immunization services, and safety-engineered injection devices, including reuse prevention (RUP) syringes and sharps injury prevention (SIP) devices for therapeutic injections *(31)* (http://apps.who.int/iris/bitstream/10665/44102/1/9789241597906_eng.pdf); (http://www.who.int/bloodsafety/publications/UniversalAccesstoSafeBT.pdf?ua=1); (http://www.euro.who.int/__data/assets/pdf_file/0005/268790/WHO-guidelines-on-drawing-blood-best-practices-in-phlebotomy-Eng.pdf?ua=1).

2. GUIDING PRINCIPLES

2.1. Promoting human rights and equity in access to hepatitis testing

Access to health care is a basic human right and applies equally to men, women and children, regardless of gender, race, sexual preference, socioeconomic status or behavioural practices, including drug use, and is in keeping with the United Nations Universal Declaration of Human Rights *(32)*. The promotion of human rights and equity in access to hepatitis B and C testing, prevention, treatment and care are guiding principles central to these guidelines. Persons with hepatitis B and C infection may come from vulnerable groups because of low socioeconomic status with poor access to appropriate health care, or because they belong to groups that are marginalized or stigmatized such as PWID, MSM, migrants, indigenous peoples or prisoners. Hepatitis testing services need to ensure that testing is accessible to the populations most affected, and that these groups are offered testing in an environment that minimizes stigma and discrimination. Informed consent should always be obtained. Screening for viral hepatitis must not be used as a means to discriminate against those testing positive. The provision of adequate safeguards to ensure confidentiality, and a non-coercive approach are fundamental principles of good clinical practice.

2.2. The public health approach along the continuum of care

In accordance with existing WHO guidance on HIV testing *(11)*, use of antiretrovirals (ARVs) *(23),* and HBV and HCV treatment *(6, 5)*, these guidelines are based on a public health approach to scaling up testing and treatment for hepatitis B and C across the entire continuum of care. The public health approach seeks to ensure the widest possible access to high-quality services at the population level, based on simplified and standardized approaches that can readily be taken to scale and decentralized, including in resource-limited settings. A public health approach aims to strike a balance between implementing the best-proven standard of care and what is feasible on a large scale in resource-limited settings, and to achieve health equity, promote gender equality, engage communities, and leverage public and private sectors in the response.

2.3. The WHO "5 Cs"

The WHO "5 Cs" are principles that apply to all models of hepatitis testing and in all settings: Consent, Confidentiality, Counselling, Correct test results and Connection (linkage to prevention, treatment and care services) *(11)*. This means hepatitis testing for diagnosis must always be voluntary, and consent for testing informed by pre-test information. Testing should be linked to prevention, treatment, care and support services to maximize both individual and public health benefits. Mandatory, compulsory or coercive hepatitis testing is never appropriate, whether that coercion comes from a health-care provider, an employer, authorities (such as immigration services) or a partner or family member. All testing sites should ensure client confidentiality.

2.4. Accurate testing

Patients have the right to accurate and high quality testing to ensure that those requiring treatment are identified and initiated, while those who are negative or not in need of treatment are not inappropriately treated. The foundation of accurate testing includes: (i) provision of reliable, high quality, regulatory approved test kits; (ii) qualified, trained, competent and supported testing personnel; and (iii) quality-assured testing environment that addresses quality (process) control, equipment management and maintenance, accurate recordkeeping and documentation (standard operating procedures (SOPs), and external quality assessment (EQA) schemes.

Some countries will face significant challenges as they seek to implement testing for chronic hepatitis B and hepatitis C infection due to constraints in resources and health systems. Each country will need to plan its own approach to implementing quality hepatitis testing services. Such services should be informed by the local context, including national hepatitis B and C epidemiology, availability of appropriately trained individuals and suitable laboratory capacity with quality management systems in place. Other considerations are efficient supply systems for laboratory commodities, availability of financial resources, organization and capacity of the health system, anticipated cost–effectiveness of the various interventions, and fair and equitable expansion in access.

3. METHODOLOGY AND PROCESS OF DEVELOPING THE GUIDELINES

3.1. WHO guideline development process

These WHO guidelines were developed following the recommendations for standard guidelines as described in the WHO *Handbook for Guideline Development (33)*, and the GRADE framework *(34–37)* (Tables 3.1, 3.2 and Box 3.1). A Guidelines Development Group was formed with representation from different geographical regions as well as from a wide range of stakeholders, including researchers, clinicians and programme managers, advocacy groups and members of organizations that represent persons living with chronic hepatitis. There was an initial scoping and planning process to formulate questions most relevant to LMICs and patient-important outcomes (*see Web annex 4* for all PICO questions).

3.2. Systematic reviews and additional background work

Systematic reviews on diagnostic performance. Systematic reviews and meta-analyses of the primary literature were commissioned externally to address the research questions and patient-important outcomes. For evaluation of HBV and HCV diagnostics and testing strategies, there was very limited or no evidence for patient-important outcomes. The Guidelines Development Group and PICO questions considered diagnostic accuracy (sensitivity, specificity, positive and negative predictive values) and in some cases analytical sensitivity (limit of detection) as surrogates for patient-important outcomes, assuming reasonable linkage and access to care. Search strategies and summaries of evidence are reported in *Web annex 5*. The glossary provides full definitions for diagnostic and analytical test performance.

As part of the guidelines development process, WHO commissioned other work to provide additional data to support the recommendations. These are given below.

• **Existing systematic reviews on global and regional seroprevalence** of HBsAg and HCV antibody in general population and **specific high-risk populations** (Table 4.1).

• **Review of the cost–effectiveness literature of different viral hepatitis testing approaches in different settings.** The evidence base for different testing approaches remains very limited, especially for impact on patient-important outcomes and in LMICs, and largely relies on observational data and modelling.

The limited number of cost–effectiveness studies and the heterogeneity of study populations, testing approaches and outcomes measured precluded a formal systematic review and meta-analysis. A narrative review was therefore undertaken that included studies of: (i) focused or targeted testing of the highest-risk groups; (ii) routine testing among specific birth cohorts that are readily identified and have a high prevalence of HCV infection; and (iii) routine testing throughout the entire population, in different settings.

• **Predictive modelling** of testing strategies (i.e. one- or two-test serological testing strategies). There were very few studies that directly compared different testing strategies for diagnostic accuracy and therefore a predictive modelling analysis was carried out to examine the accuracy of a testing strategy across a range of performance characteristics of the assays (sensitivity and specificity) based on the systematic reviews, and a hypothetical range of prevalence of the disease in the population (10%, 2%, 0.4%) representing high-, medium- and low-prevalence settings or populations (*see Web annex 6*).

• **Values and preferences survey of health-care workers and implementers for different testing strategies and approaches.** A four-part online survey tool was undertaken in September 2015, which covered questions on current and preferences for future HBV and HCV testing practices, including a test of HCV cure. Respondents included clinicians, patient organizations, civil society representatives, programme managers, policy-makers and pharmaceutical industry employees.

• **Feasibility survey** on programmatic experiences and reports of barriers/challenges to HBV and/or HCV testing based on 22 interviewees across 13 LMICs conducted between June and September 2015. The 33-question semi-structured questionnaire covered programme information (who is tested and where, what assays/algorithms are used, counselling and training, funding and costs of testing); protocol for hepatitis care and treatment; perceived barriers/challenges and solutions; and provision of relevant epidemiological data.

• **Case examples of different models of hepatitis testing practices in different settings and populations** were also solicited and identified through a hepatitis testing innovation contest, to illustrate effective and acceptable ways to deliver facility and community-based testing services, especially among most affected populations.

3.3. Grading of quality of evidence and strength of recommendations

The quality of the evidence was assessed and either rated down or rated up based on criteria specified in GRADE methods, modified for diagnostic tests and test strategies *(38, 39)*. Summaries of the quality of evidence to address each outcome were entered in the GRADE profiler software (GRADE pro 3.6). The quality of evidence was categorized as high, moderate, low or very low (Box 3.1 and Table 3.1).

Specific issues with rating quality of evidence for studies of diagnostic accuracy and strategies

Diagnostic test accuracy. For evaluation of HBV and HCV diagnostics and testing strategies, there was very limited or no evidence on effects on patient-important outcomes. The Guidelines Development Group and PICO questions considered diagnostic accuracy (sensitivity, specificity, positive and negative predictive values) and in some cases analytical sensitivity (limit of detection) as surrogates for patient-important outcomes, assuming reasonable linkage and access to care.

Although observational studies of interventions start as low quality in GRADE, cross-sectional and cohort studies of diagnostic accuracy can provide reliable evidence *(38)*, and were therefore initially categorized as high quality. Evidence was then rated down based on the presence of (i) risk of bias (using a tool designed for assessment of diagnostic accuracy studies, the QUADAS-2 tool) *(40)*; (ii) inconsistency or heterogeneity; (iii) indirectness (addressing a different population than the one under consideration); or (iv) imprecision. However, evaluating inconsistency in studies of diagnostic accuracy is a challenge because methods to measure statistical heterogeneity are lacking and inconsistency is common, and therefore we did not downgrade for indirectness.

Testing strategies. Clinical studies to evaluate comparisons of different testing strategies and approaches were generally not available. Therefore, the Guidelines Development Group considered instead predictive modelling to generate estimates of diagnostic performance of different testing strategies. This type of evidence was not formally graded but was considered low quality because it is very indirect.

BOX 3.1. Standard approach to rating the quality of evidence and strength of recommendations using the GRADE system

The GRADE system separates the rating of the quality of evidence from the rating of the strength of the recommendation.

The **quality of evidence** is defined as the confidence that the reported estimates of effect are adequate to support a specific recommendation. The GRADE system classifies the quality of evidence as high, moderate, low and very low *(35, 37, 41–45)*. For studies of interventions, randomized controlled trials (RCTs) are initially rated as high-quality evidence but may be downgraded for several reasons, including the risk of bias, inconsistency of results across studies, indirectness of evidence, imprecision and publication bias. Observational studies of interventions are initially rated as low-quality evidence but may be upgraded if the magnitude of the treatment effect is very large, if multiple studies show the same effect, if evidence indicates a dose–response relationship, or if all plausible biases would underestimate the effect *(41)*. The higher the quality of evidence, the more likely a strong recommendation can be made.

The **strength of a recommendation** reflects the extent to which the Guidelines Development Group was confident that the desirable effects of following a recommendation outweigh the potential undesirable effects. The GRADE system classifies the strength of a recommendation in two ways: "strong" and "conditional" *(37)*. The strength is influenced by the following factors: the quality of the evidence, balance of benefits and harms, values and preferences, resource use and the feasibility of carrying out the intervention (Table 3.2).

A strong recommendation is one for which the Guidelines Development Group was confident that the desirable effects of adhering to the recommendation outweigh the undesirable effects.

A conditional recommendation is one for which the Guidelines Development Group concluded that the desirable effects of adhering to the recommendation probably outweigh the undesirable effects but the Guidelines Development Group is not confident about these trade-offs. The implications of a conditional recommendation are that, although most people or settings would adopt the recommendation, many would not or would do so only under certain conditions. The reasons for making a conditional recommendation include the absence of high-quality evidence, imprecision in outcome estimates, uncertainty regarding how individuals value the outcomes, small benefits relative to harms, and benefits that may not be worth the costs (including the costs of implementing the recommendation).

TABLE 3.1. GRADE categories of the quality of evidence

Level of evidence	Rationale
High	Further research is very unlikely to change our confidence in the estimate of effect.
Moderate	Further research is likely to have an important impact on our confidence in the effect.
Low	Further research is very likely to have an estimate of effect and is likely to change the estimate.
Very low	Any estimate of effect is very uncertain.

TABLE 3.2. Key domains considered in determining the strength of recommendations

Domain	Rationale
Benefits and risks/harms	Desirable effects (benefits) need to be weighed against undesirable effects (risks/harms). The more the benefits outweigh the risks, the more likely a strong recommendation will be made.
Values and preferences (acceptability)	If the recommendation is likely to be widely accepted or highly valued, a strong recommendation will probably be made. If there are strong reasons that the recommended course of action is unlikely to be accepted, a conditional recommendation is more likely to be made.
Costs and financial implications (resource use)	Lower costs (monetary, infrastructure, equipment or human resources) or greater cost–effectiveness will more likely result in a strong recommendation.
Feasibility	If an intervention is achievable in a setting where the greatest impact is expected, a strong recommendation is more probable.

3.4. Formulation of recommendations

At the September 2015 meeting of the Guidelines Development Group, for each of the PICO questions (*see Web annex 4*), the results of the systematic reviews and the evidence profiles (*see Web annexes 5* and *6*) were presented and reviewed. Commissioned surveys of diagnostic costs, values and preferences for different testing strategies of health-care workers and implementing partners, and a global survey of programmatic experience were also considered. Recommendations were then formulated based on the overall quality of the evidence, in addition to other considerations, including the balance between benefits and harms, values and preferences, feasibility and resource implications (Table 3.2). The strength of the recommendations was rated as either strong (the panel was confident that the benefits of the intervention outweighed the risks) or conditional (the panel considered that the benefits of the intervention outweighed the risks, but the balance of benefits to harms and burdens was small or uncertain). Recommendations were then formulated and the wording finalized by the entire Group. Implementation needs were subsequently evaluated, and areas and topics requiring further research identified.

For recommendations based on diagnostic accuracy, the Guidelines Development Group considered potential trade-offs between diagnostic accuracy and other factors. Although diagnostic accuracy was considered a critical outcome and a reasonable surrogate for patient outcomes, tests and testing strategies associated with slightly lower diagnostic accuracy could be recommended when associated with lower costs, increased testing access and linkage to care or greater feasibility.

3.5. Declaration and management of conflicts of interest

In accordance with WHO policy, all members of the Guidelines Development Group and peer reviewers were required to complete and submit a WHO Declaration of Interest form (including participation in consulting and advisory panels, research support and financial investment) and, where appropriate, also provide a summary of research interests and activities. The WHO Secretariat then reviewed and assessed the declarations submitted by each member and, at the September 2015 meeting of the Guidelines Development Group, presented a summary to the Guidelines Development Group (*see Web annex 7*). The WHO Secretariat stated that there had been a transparent declaration of financial and academic interests, and concluded that there were no conflicts that required exclusion of any member from actively taking part in formulating the recommendations during the meeting. For the peer review group, the WHO Secretariat was also satisfied that no case necessitated exclusion from the review process.

3.6. Updating, disseminating and monitoring implementation of the guidelines

The guidelines are accessible on the WHO website with links to other related websites, and translated into the official United Nations (UN) languages. WHO disseminates the guidelines to ministries of health in countries, as well as key international, regional and national collaborating partners (e.g. civil society, foundations, donors).

Successful implementation of these guidelines will be assessed by the number of countries that incorporate the contents into national hepatitis plans and guidelines. The impact of the testing guidelines will be measured by monitoring the number of persons tested and treated for chronic hepatitis B and hepatitis C infection, in accordance with targets proposed in the WHO *Global health sector strategy on viral hepatitis 2016–2021 (16) (*see Web annex 1)*. The Guidelines Development Group recognized that the field of hepatitis diagnostics and testing is evolving rapidly, and it is anticipated that there will be a need for periodic updates.

4. BACKGROUND – EPIDEMIOLOGY AND NATURAL HISTORY

An understanding of the global and regional epidemiology and burden of hepatitis B and C infection with respect to the main routes of transmission, most affected populations, and natural history and time course of serological markers is critical to inform strategies on both who to test and how to test. However, data are limited in many LMICs, particularly in the African region, due to weak surveillance systems with underreporting and therefore unreliable data. The nature of an epidemic within a specific country will determine the appropriate testing strategy and approaches. Table 4.1 provides an overview of the risk factors and primary routes of transmission for HBV and HCV infection in populations most affected by HBV and HCV, as well as data on seroprevalence from systematic reviews and other studies.

TABLE 4.1. Overview of populations most affected by HBV and HCV infection with summary of risk factors, primary routes of transmission and seroprevalence rates

Key and priority populations	Hepatitis B	Hepatitis C
People who inject drugs (PWID)	High risk of infection through parenteral exposure, most commonly from sharing of needles and other injecting equipment.	
	Prevalence rates of HBV infection among PWID similar to background population in HBV-endemic areas (1, 46, 47)	Global prevalence estimated to be 67% among PWID in 77 countries and over 80% in 12 countries) (46). Prevalence is particularly high in settings where PWID are criminalized and lack access to harm reduction services.
		Non-injecting drug use, e.g. through intranasal drug use, has been associated with a small but increased risk of HCV infection (48).
People in prisons and closed settings	High risk of infection through parenteral exposure, most commonly from sharing of needles and razor blades and other injecting equipment, particularly when safe injecting equipment is not available (25, 49).	
	Potential for increased risk of sexual transmission due to unsafe sex behaviours, lack of availability of prevention hardware such as condoms, and higher risk of experiencing men-on-men sexual violence (50)	
		Estimated global prevalence ranges from 23% to 29%, with rates as high as 40% reported from some regions, including Australia, North America, western Europe, Central Asia, East and South-East Asia (51)

Key and priority populations	Hepatitis B	Hepatitis C
Mobile or migrant populations	Migrants from intermediate- and high-endemic HBV areas are at increased risk of chronic hepatitis B (CHB) *(52–54)*.	Migrant populations represent a heterogeneous group and HCV seroprevalence estimates vary widely *(52–54)*.
	Displaced and marginalized populations may be at increased risk of sexual transmission of HBV due to increased vulnerability to sexual violence or coercion, or unsafe sex practices *(53, 54)*.	
	Some marginalized mobile populations may be more likely to belong to other populations at high risk for HBV and HCV transmission, such as PWID or sex workers *(53, 54)*.	
Indigenous populations	Some indigenous populations may have higher rates of prevalence but poorer access to HBV vaccination or be more likely to belong to other high-risk populations, such as PWID *(55, 56)*.	Some indigenous populations may be more likely to belong to other high-risk populations, such as PWID *(55, 56)*.
Sex workers	Sex workers are at increased risk of sexual transmission of HBV due to exposure to multiple partners and poorer access to access safe sex materials such as condoms *(56)*.	Overall, the risk of sexual transmission of HCV is low. There may be a small, increased risk of transmission among persons with multiple sex partners.
	Sex workers may be more likely to belong to other high-risk populations, such as PWID and persons in prisons or closed settings *(56)*.	
Transgender people	Transgender people may be at increased risk for viral hepatitis through using unsafe injecting equipment for administration of hormones or through sexual transmission *(57)*.	
Men who have sex with men (MSM)	MSM are at increased risk of sexual acquisition of HBV *(58)*.	Risk of sexual transmission of HCV is low among HIV-negative MSM. HIV-positive MSM are at significantly increased risk of sexual transmission of HCV, particularly those who engage in high-risk sex behaviours such as unprotected anal sex *(59–63)*.
		In several outbreaks of HCV infection among MSM in Europe, Australia and the US, transmission has been linked to sexual exposure as well as potentially to underreported use of injecting and non-injecting recreational drugs *(63–65)*.

Key and priority populations	Hepatitis B	Hepatitis C
Health-care workers	The greatest proportion of occupational transmission of viral hepatitis is due to percutaneous injury via needles during vascular access. Transmission may also occur through exposure to blood and body fluids on skin lesions and mucous membranes *(66)*.	
	Multiple factors contribute to higher risk of occupational acquisition in LMICs. These include: working among populations with a higher prevalence of infection, higher rates of unnecessary injections in health-care settings, use of unsterilized needles and equipment lacking a needle-stick safety mechanism, lack of implementation of standard precautions, inadequate coverage of HBV vaccination *(67)*.	
	Among non-immune persons, the risk of HBV infection after percutaneous exposure ranges from less than 6% (if HBeAg negative) to 30% (if HBeAg posiitive) *(68)*.	Risk of HCV infection after percutaneous exposure estimated to be 1.8% *(68)*.
Persons exposed in health-care settings	High risk of parenteral transmission in settings with a higher background seroprevalence of HBV and HCV and where infection control practices are inadequate (e.g. diagnostic and therapeutic procedures), and blood transfusions and other tissue donations are not screened for viral hepatitis *(69–79)*.	
	Persons who may have multiple exposures, such as patients with thalassaemia or haemophilia who receive multiple transfusions, and patients on haemodialysis, are at higher risk *(80–82)*.	
Persons exposed via other invasive procedures	There is a small but increased risk of HBV and HCV transmission with other procedures where there is a risk blood-to-blood transmission via contaminated equipment, including cosmetic procedures (such as tattooing and body piercing), and traditional medicine procedures such as scarification and circumcision *(80–82)*.	
Persons living with HIV and those living with other sexually transmitted infections (STIs)	Persons who have been exposed to HIV or other STIs via sexual transmission may be at increased risk of sexually acquired HBV infection *(87)*.	There is an increased risk of HCV infection among persons living with HIV *(88–93)*.
	Particularly in high HBV and HCV-prevalence settings, children who have been exposed to HIV through mother-to-child transmission (MTCT) are at increased risk of HBV and HCV infection *(86)*.	
Infants born to infected mothers	Perinatal or early childhood transmission is the main route of infection in many parts of the world, particularly in endemic countries, where 90% of CHB infections may be attributable to MTCT.	MTCT is the most common cause of HCV infection in young children. Risk of HCV transmission is 4–8% in the perinatal period, and 10%–25% among children born to mothers coinfected with HIV *(96–99)*.
	HBV transmission in early life is associated with a much higher risk of developing chronic infection (90% in the perinatal period to 6 months of age) than acquisition later in childhood or adulthood) *(94, 95)*.	

Key and priority populations	Hepatitis B	Hepatitis C
Children	Horizontal (household, intra-familial and child-to-child) transmission is an important route of infection. Up to 50% of childhood CHB infections cannot be accounted for by MTCT of HBV.	Based on limited data, horizontal transmission does not appear to be a significant contributor to HCV transmission in children *(100)*. High prevalence in some settings such as in children treated in hospital for malignancy, renal failure requiring haemodialysis, and those who have undergone surgical procedures likely reflects iatrogenic transmission *(101)*.
Adolescents	There may also be adolescents who missed out on HBV vaccination, and were infected perinatally or in early childhood. Adolescents who engage in early sex, have multiple sex partners, or sex partners with CHB are at increased risk *(25)*.	Overall, the risk of sexual transmission of HCV is low. However, there is a small increased risk among persons with multiple sex partners *(59, 102)*.
	Vulnerable adolescents may be more likely to belong to other high-risk key populations, including PWID and sex workers, for example *(25)*.	
Couples, partners and household contacts	Persons who live in the same household as a person with CHB are at increased risk of horizontal acquisition of HBV infection *(103)*.	Overall, the risk of sexual transmission of HCV is low. However, the risk is increased among persons with multiple sex partners *(59, 102, 104)*. There is no evidence to support transmission among household contacts who are not sexual partners *(100)*.

CHB: chronic hepatitis B; HBeAg: hepatitis B e antigen; HBsAg: hepatitis B surface antigen; HBV: hepatitis B virus; HCV: hepatitis C virus; insert MTCT: mother-to-child transmission; MSM: men who have sex with men; PWID: people who inject drugs; STI: sexually transmitted infection

4.1. Hepatitis B infection

4.1.1. Epidemiology of hepatitis B infection

It is estimated that worldwide, 2 billion people have evidence of past or present infection with HBV, and 248 million are chronic carriers of HBV surface antigen (HBsAg), particularly in LMICs *(2)*. Age-specific HBsAg seroprevalence varies markedly by geographical region, with the highest prevalence (>5%) in sub-Saharan Africa (SSA), east Asia, some parts of the Balkan region, the Pacific Islands and Amazon Basin of South America. Prevalence below 2% is seen in regions such as Central America, North America and Western Europe *(2)*. Overall, almost half of the global population lives in areas of high and intermediate endemicity.

The major complications of CHB are cirrhosis and HCC. Worldwide, it is estimated that around 686 000 people die each year from the complications of CHB *(1)*. Overall, HBV infection accounts for around 45% of cases of HCC and 30% of cirrhosis, with much higher proportions in LMICs *(1, 105)*. In Asia and most other regions, the incidence of HCC and cirrhosis is low before the age of 35–40 years but then rises exponentially *(1)*. However, in some parts of Africa, Alaska and the Amazon, the incidence of HCC is also high in infected children and young adult men *(106)*.

HIV and HBV. There is an estimated global HBsAg prevalence of 7·4% (IQR 5.0– 11.2%) in HIV-infected persons, and a burden of 2.73 million (IQR 1.8–3.9 million; IQR 1·3–4·4 million) HIV–HBsAg-coinfected persons *(87)*. The highest burden for HIV–HBV coinfection is in sub-Saharan Africa (SSA) (71% of all cases; 1.96 million).

4.1.2. Transmission of hepatitis B infection

Table 4.1 provides an overview of the risk factors and primary routes of transmission for HBV infection in populations most affected by hepatitis B. HBV is spread predominantly by percutaneous or mucosal exposure to infected blood and various body fluids, including saliva and menstrual, vaginal and seminal fluids. Perinatal transmission is the major route of HBV transmission in many parts of the world, and an important factor in maintaining the reservoir of the infection in some regions, particularly in China and South-East Asia *(107, 108)*. Horizontal transmission, including household, interfamilial and especially child to child, is also important *(103)*. Both sexual and oral transmission of hepatitis B may occur, particularly in unvaccinated MSM and heterosexual persons with multiple sex partners or contact with sex workers. Transmission of the virus may also result from accidental inoculation of minute amounts of blood or fluid during medical, surgical and dental procedures, or from razors and similar objects contaminated with infected blood; immunization with inadequately sterilized syringes and needles; injecting drug use; tattooing; body piercing; and acupuncture. Unvaccinated health-care workers are also at risk of accidental transmission of hepatitis B during handling contaminated sharps, body fluids and organs, and medical waste.

4.1.3. Natural history of HBV infection

Hepatitis B virus is an enveloped DNA virus, and a member of the family *Hepadnaviridae* hepatotropic DNA viruses. Hepatitis B virus causes both acute and chronic infection that can range from asymptomatic infection or mild disease to severe or fulminant hepatitis. **Acute hepatitis B** is usually a self-limiting disease marked by acute inflammation and hepatocellular necrosis, with a case fatality rate of 0.5–1% *(109)*. **Chronic hepatitis B (CHB)** encompasses a spectrum of disease, and is defined as persistent HBV infection (the presence of detectable HBsAg in the blood or serum for longer than six months), with or without associated active viral replication and evidence of hepatocellular injury and inflammation *(109)*. Age is a key factor in determining the risk of chronic infection. Chronicity is common following acute infection in neonates (90% of neonates born to hepatitis B e antigen [HBeAg]-positive mothers) and in young children under the age of 5 years (20–60%), but occurs less commonly (<5%) when infection is acquired in adulthood *(94, 95)* (Fig. 4.1). Worldwide, the majority of persons with CHB were infected at birth or in early childhood.

FIG. 4.1 Outcomes of hepatitis B virus infection by age at infection

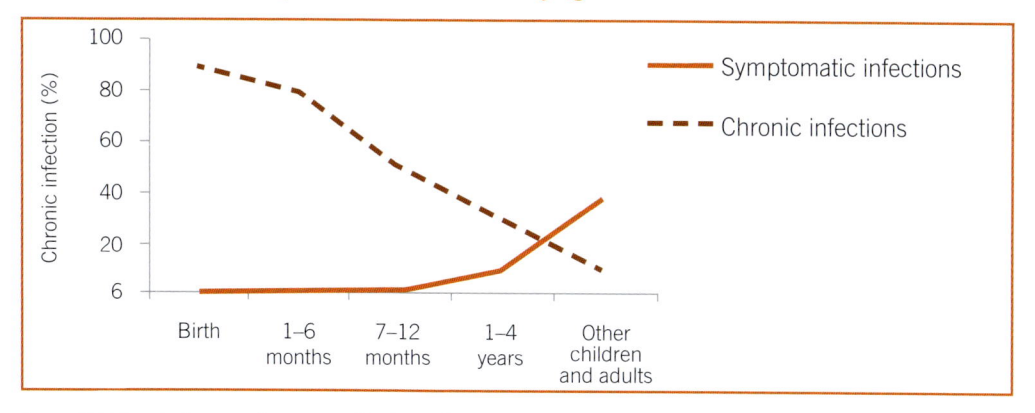

Source: Guidelines for the prevention, care and treatment of persons with hepatitis B infection. Geneva: WHO; 2015 (http://www.who.int/hepatitis/publications/hepatitis-b-guidelines/en/, accessed 15 June 2016) *(6)*.

The natural history of CHB is dynamic and complex, and progresses non-linearly through several recognizable phases *(6, 95)*. The phases are of variable duration, not necessarily sequential, and do not always relate directly to criteria and indications for antiviral therapy *(47)*.

4.1.4. Time course and interpretation of serological markers of HBV infection

A range of HBV markers other than HBsAg, such as anti-HBc total and anti-HBc IgM, HBeAg and antibodies to hepatitis B e and surface antigen (anti-HBe and anti-HBs) and HBV DNA can be used to further characterize HBV infection (*see* Table 4.2). When these markers are tested concurrently, a testing profile can be produced to differentiate acute from chronic infection, stage the disease and identify those who may benefit from treatment, monitor disease progression or response to antiviral treatment, as well as those who would benefit from HBV immunization or re-immunization.

The appearance of HBsAg in the blood is followed by that of HBeAg, which is a marker of high levels of viral replication. In acute HBV infection that resolves by itself, HBeAg seroconverts relatively early to anti-HBe with the disappearance of HBsAg and HBeAg. But in chronic HBV infection, seroconversion to anti-HBe may be delayed for many years, HBeAg may persist, or neither anti-HBe nor HBeAg may be detectable in the presence of HBsAg. Antibodies to hepatitis B core antigen (anti-HBc) may occur relatively early in the infection, often within a week or two after the appearance of HBsAg, and is typified by a profound immunoglobulin (Ig)M anti-HBc response that wanes approximately 6 months later (Fig. 4.2 and 4.3).

FIG. 4.2 Acute HBV infection with recovery

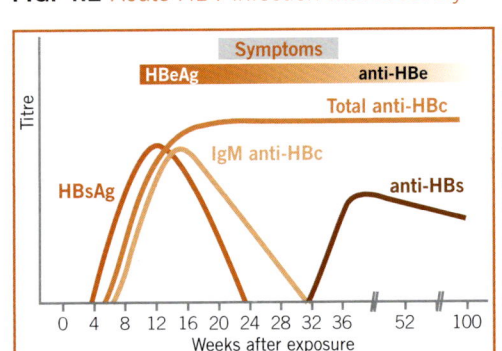

FIG. 4.3 Chronic HBV infection

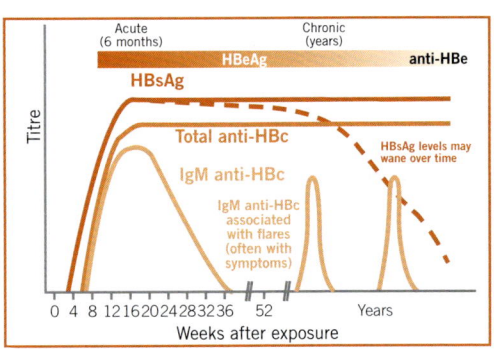

CHB is defined as the persistence of HBsAg for more than 6 months. Previous HBV infection is characterized by the presence of antibodies (anti-HBs and anti-HBc). Immunity to HBV infection after vaccination is characterized by the presence of only anti-HBs.

It also needs to be established whether the person is in the HBeAg-positive or HBeAg-negative phase of infection, though both require lifelong monitoring, as the condition may change over time. In persons with CHB, a positive HBeAg result suggests high-level HBV replication and high infectivity. Spontaneous improvement may occur following HBeAg-positive seroconversion (anti-HBe), with a decline in HBV replication, and normalization of alanine aminotransferase (ALT) levels. This confers a good prognosis and does not require treatment.

Further assessment of HBsAg-positive persons is needed to guide management and indicate the need for treatment *(6)*. This generally includes assessment of additional serological markers of HBV infection (HBeAg), measuring aminotransferase levels to help determine liver inflammation, quantification of HBV DNA levels, and stage of liver fibrosis by non-invasive tests (NITs) such as transient elastography or serum biomarker-based tests such as aspartate aminotransferase (AST)-to-platelet ratio index (APRI), and fibrosis-4 (FIB-4).

TABLE 4.2. Summary of markers of HBV infection

Marker	Characteristics
HBsAg	• First serological marker of HBV infection to appear (Fig. 4.2 & 4.3) • Window period between HBV infection and detection of HBsAg estimated to be around 38 days, but depends on analytical sensitivity of assay used, immunocompetence of host and individual virus kinetics • Occult HBV infection[a] has been observed, i.e. HBsAg is undetectable but HBV DNA can be detected in individuals not in the window period • Quantification of HBsAg[b] is a potential alternative marker of viraemia and to monitor response to antiviral treatment

Marker	Characteristics
Anti-HBc IgM[c]	• High levels present during acute infection but may remain detectable for up to 6 months • Used to differentiate between acute and chronic HBV infection, but its reappearance during "flares" in chronic HBV infection make it an unreliable indicator of recent primary HBV infection (Fig. 4.3)
Anti-HBc (total)	• Develops around 3 months after infection and most constant marker of infection • Together with anti-HBs, indicates resolved infection • Anti-HBc, with or without anti-HBs, also indicates individuals who may reactivate in the context of immunosuppression
HBeAg	• Present when the virus is actively replicating in the liver • Associated with high levels of HBV viraemia and is therefore a marker of "high infectivity" • Associated with progressive liver disease
Anti-HBe	• Represents host response to HBeAg and usually indicates decreasing HBV DNA and therefore infectivity • Present in the immune-control and immune-escape phases • May coexist with HBeAg during the period of seroconversion from e antigen to e antibody at the end of immune-tolerance phase
Anti-HBs	• Neutralizing antibody that confers protection from infection • Present following spontaneous HBsAg clearance (with anti-HBc IgG) • Generated by immunization and used to monitor post-immunization responses (anti-HBc absent) • May coexist with HBsAg so presence cannot be used to exclude current infection
HBV DNA	• Used as a more direct and accurate measure of active HBV viral replication, which correlates with disease progression • Serum HBV DNA is measured in international units (IU)/mL[d] as the recognized international standard or copies/ml by nucleic acid testing (NAT) technologies • Used to differentiate active from inactive HBeAg-negative, and to determine need for antiviral therapy in conjunction with ALT levels and degree of liver fibrosis • Used to also monitor response to therapy (a rise may indicate inadequate adherence or the emergence of resistant variants) and as a marker of infectivity. • May be detectable in early infection before HBsAg, and therefore useful in early diagnosis of at-risk individuals before HBsAg appears, but depends on sensitivity of the assay • Also present at low levels in the absence of HBsAg in the context of occult infection

anti-HBc: antibody to hepatitis B core antigen; anti-HBs: antibody to hepatitis B surface antigen; HBeAg: hepatitis B e antigen; HBsAg: hepatitis B surface antigen; Ig: immunoglobulin

[a] Occult HBV infection: HBsAg is undetectable while HBV DNA can be detected in individuals who are not in the window period; mostly anti-HBc is also detectable. Evidence of onward transmission of occult HBV infection has been indicated in the literature, but impact on morbidity and/or mortality is less well described.

[b] However, as most antivirals used to treat HBV block DNA replication pathways (by inhibiting reverse transcription) rather than transcription/translation HBsAg pathways, HBsAg levels are minimally impacted by antivirals.

[c] A potential consequence of misinterpreting a reactive IgM anti-HBc result is that a patient with chronic HBV infection experiencing flares in liver disease may not be offered timely antiviral treatment and, although they could be re-examined several months later to confirm the original diagnosis of acute HBV infection, a substantial proportion of such patients may be lost to follow up.

[d] 1 IU/mL = 5.3 copies/mL; 2000 IU/mL = 10 000 copies/mL; 20 000 IU/mL = 100 000 copies/mL; 200 000 IU/mL = 1 000 000 copies/mL

4.1.5. Preventing hepatitis B infection through vaccination

Vaccination of infants and, in particular, delivery of hepatitis B vaccine within 24 hours of birth is 90–95% effective in preventing infection with HBV as well as in decreasing HBV transmission if followed by at least two other doses. WHO recommends universal hepatitis B vaccination for all infants, and giving the first dose as soon as possible after birth *(24)*. This strategy has resulted in a dramatic decrease in the incidence and prevalence of CHB among young children in regions of the world where universal infant vaccination programmes have been implemented *(110, 111)*. Target groups for catch-up vaccination as well as other preventive strategies include young adolescents, household and sexual contacts of persons who are HBsAg-positive, and persons at risk of acquiring HBV infection, such as PWID, MSM and persons with multiple sex partners.

4.1.6. Treatment of hepatitis B infection

WHO recommends antiviral agents (tenofovir and entecavir) that are active against HBV infection and have been shown to effectively suppress HBV replication, prevent progression to cirrhosis, and reduce the risk of HCC and liver-related deaths *(6, 112, 113)*. However, in the majority of patients, treatment with these drugs does not provide cure (i.e. the person continues to have replicating virus), necessitating potentially lifelong treatment.

4.2. Hepatitis C infection

4.2.1. Epidemiology of hepatitis C infection

Recent analyses of the global prevalence of HCV indicate that there may be fewer persons living with hepatitis C infection than previously estimated. A recent systematic review estimated that 110 million persons have a history of HCV infection (i.e. are HCV-antibody positive) and 80 million have chronic viraemic infection *(3)*. Regions estimated to have a high prevalence in the general population (>3.5%) are Central and east Asia, and North Africa/Middle East; those with a moderate prevalence (1.5–3.5%) include South and South-East Asia, Sub-Saharan Africa, Latin America (Andean, central, and southern regions), the Caribbean, Oceania, Australasia, and central, eastern and western Europe; whereas low-prevalence (<1.5%) regions include Asia–Pacific, Latin America, and North America *(3)*. Updated estimates in Africa show a HCV prevalence of 2.98%, with a higher prevalence observed in west Africa and lower in south-east Africa *(114)*.

Despite the declining incidence, a large number of persons who were infected 30–60 years ago are now dying from HCV-related cirrhosis and liver cancer, as these complications often take decades to develop. According to estimates from the Global Burden of Disease study, the number of deaths due to hepatitis C increased from 333 000 in 1990 to 499 000 in 2010 and 704 000 in 2013 *(1, 5, 115)*, and this increase is projected to continue for several more decades, unless treatment is scaled up considerably *(116)*.

HIV and HCV have common routes of transmission, and persons with HIV infection, in particular PWID and MSM, are at increased risk of HCV infection *(60, 62, 88–93, 117)*. In a recent comprehensive systematic review, it is estimated that, globally, 2.3 million persons are coinfected with these two viruses, of whom 1.2 million (interquartile range [IQR] 0.9–1.4 million) are PWID *(88)*. With the widespread use of antiretroviral therapy (ART), which reduces the risk of HIV-associated opportunistic infections, HCV-related liver disease has started to overtake AIDS-defining illnesses as a leading cause of death among people living with HIV in some high-income countries (HICs) *(118)*.

4.2.2. Transmission of hepatitis C infection

Table 4.1 provides an overview of the primary routes of transmission for HCV infection and populations most affected. There are four main routes of transmission: **health-care-associated transmission, injecting drug use, mother-to-child transmission (MTCT), and sexual transmission.** In LMICs, infection with HCV is most commonly associated with unsafe injection practices, and invasive procedures in health-care facilities with inadequate infection control practices, such as renal dialysis and unscreened (or inadequately screened) blood transfusions *(70–74, 77, 78, 119)*. Persons who received untested blood products prior to the introduction of screening of blood for HCV in (HICs) are also at risk, and WHO reports suggest that there are still 39 countries that do not routinely screen blood transfusions for bloodborne viruses *(120)*. In middle- and high-income countries, most HCV infections occur among people who use unsterile equipment to inject drugs. PWID have a high global prevalence of infection at around 67% *(46)*. Of the estimated 16 million people in 148 countries who actively inject drugs, 10 million have serological evidence of HCV infection *(46)*. There is a moderate risk of MTCT of HCV which is higher in HIV-coinfected mothers (10–20%) *(96)*. The risk of sexual transmission of HCV is also greater in HIV-positive persons, particularly MSM *(88)*, but is low among HIV-uninfected heterosexual couples *(102, 121)* and MSM *(122, 123)*. Other routes of bloodborne transmission include acquisition by health-care workers, cosmetic procedures (such as tattooing and body piercing), scarification and circumcision *(84, 85, 124)*, and intranasal drug use.

As a result of these different routes of transmission, certain groups are at higher risk of HCV infection (Table 4.1). The relative importance of these risk groups varies substantially, depending on the geographical location and population studied. Persons at risk for HCV infection are also likely to be at risk for infection with other bloodborne viruses, including HBV and HIV. Generally, HCV epidemics around the world are heterogeneous and represent mixtures of three core epidemic components (Box 4.1). However, few countries have epidemics that fall into just one of these categories – most represent some combination of all components.

Box 4.1. Global epidemic patterns of HCV infection

1. Historic infection related to past generalized HCV exposures that have since been identified and removed, i.e. "birth cohort" epidemic. These exposures include blood transfusions and medical procedures prior to the identification of HCV, or prior to the availability of HCV diagnostic screening. Following introduction of HCV screening of the blood supply in the early 1990s, the incidence of HCV fell dramatically among the general population. However, there remains a burden of prevalent, chronic HCV infection among those exposed prior to the introduction of screening of the blood supply. This epidemic pattern, in which there is a high prevalence of HCV within a given older age group, is commonly referred to as a "birth cohort" epidemic *(125)*. While typically identified as being the infection pattern in North America and Europe, it is likely to be a component of the HCV epidemic in many countries *(126)*. In addition, some countries have other specific historical risks that reflect past medical practices or public health campaigns unique to that country, for example, the use of reusable syringes in the population-based campaign to treat schistosomiasis in Egypt exposed a large proportion of the population to HCV.

2. Ongoing risk of HCV transmission reflecting current behaviours and practices

a) Ongoing infection related to high-risk behaviours. In certain countries, HCV transmission occurs predominantly in high-risk populations, often via common routes of transmission. Among PWID, HCV prevalence is almost universally high (ranging from 30% to 75% *(46)*, and in many HICs, PWID drive ongoing HCV transmission. Sex workers and prisoners also have increased prevalence (presumed to be related to both drug use and perhaps sexual transmission) *(127, 128)*, as do MSM, especially those who are HIV infected *(129)*.

b) ***Ongoing infection and generalized population epidemic related to suboptimal infection control and injection safety procedures*** in clinical settings. This pattern is related to widespread exposure, often iatrogenic, which results in high prevalence (8–10%) across all age groups. An example of a generalized exposure is the common use of reusable hypodermic syringes and needles in medical settings without adequate sterilization between uses.

The primary difference between a "birth cohort" pattern and a generalized pattern of infection is the duration of time that the generalized exposure has existed and whether it has been removed or mitigated.

FIG. 4.4 Global distribution of HCV genotypes

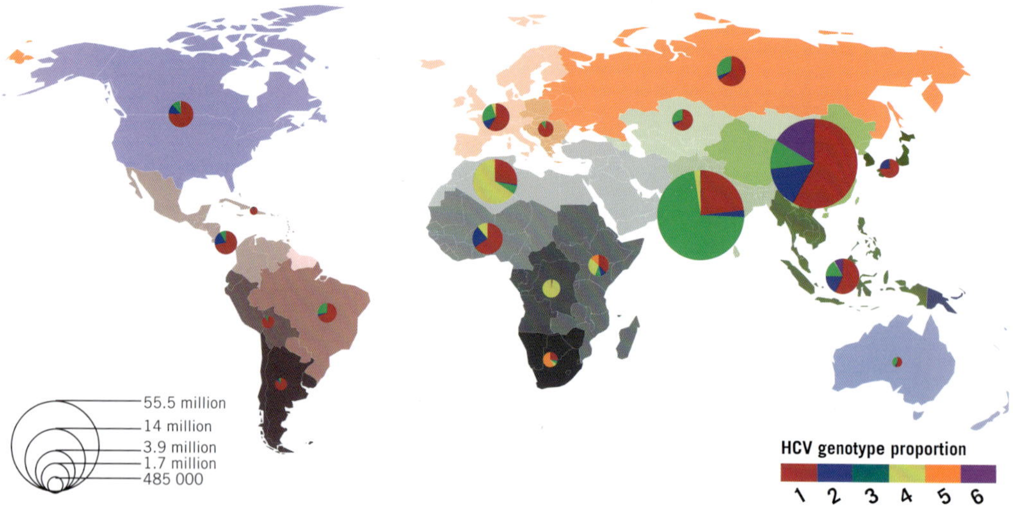

55.5 million
14 million
3.9 million
1.7 million
485 000

HCV genotype proportion
1 2 3 4 5 6

Source: Messina J.P, Humphreys I, Flaxman A, Brown A, Cooke GS, Pybus OG et al. Global distribution and prevalence of hepatitis C virus genotypes. Hepatology. 2015;77–87.

4.2.3. Natural history of hepatitis C infection

HCV is a small, positive-stranded RNA-enveloped virus with multiple genotypes and subgenotypes, and their distribution varies substantially in different parts of the world (Fig. 4.4). The availability of pangenotypic DAA regimens will increasingly obviate the need for prior genotyping, which will help expand access to HCV treatment.

Hepatitis C virus causes both acute and chronic infection. **Acute HCV infection** is defined as the presence of certain markers of HCV infection within six months of exposure to and infection with HCV, and is characterized by the appearance of HCV RNA, HCV core antigen (p22 Ag), and subsequently HCV antibodies, which may or may not be associated with viral clearance. Antibodies to HCV develop as part of acute infection and persist throughout life. Acute infection is usually clinically silent, and is only very rarely associated with life-threatening disease. Spontaneous clearance of acute HCV infection generally occurs within six months of infection in 15–45% of infected individuals in the absence of treatment, but this varies by region and population *(130)*. Antibodies to HCV develop as part of acute infection and persist throughout life. Almost all the remaining 55–85% of persons who do not clear HCV within six months are defined as having **chronic HCV infection**. Left untreated, chronic HCV infection can cause liver cirrhosis, liver failure and HCC. Of those with chronic HCV infection, the risk of cirrhosis of the liver is 15–30% within 20 years *(131–133)*. The risk of HCC in persons with cirrhosis is approximately 2–4% per year (Fig. 4.5) *(134)*. Clearance of infection, whether spontaneous or as a result of antiviral treatment, does not provide lasting protection from reinfection.

Diagnosis of HCV infection currently consists of initial screening for evidence of past or current HCV infection with a serological assay, followed by NAT for HCV RNA (either quantitative or qualitative) to confirm the presence of HCV viraemia, and therefore chronic HCV infection.

4.2.4. Time course of serological markers for HCV infection

The exact time course of virological and immunological markers of HCV infection is not well defined, particularly during the first months of infection, due to differences in each host (patient) immune response, specific properties of the infecting virus, and sensitivity of assays used to determine the appearance of HCV markers. As illustrated in Fig. 4.5, following an initial eclipse phase of 1–2 weeks when no virological or serological markers of infection may be detected, the natural course of HCV infection is characterized by the appearance of HCV RNA, then HCV core p22 Ag in the absence of an antibody response for a further 6–10 weeks. During this serological window, it has been shown that free (i.e. not complexed with antibody) HCV core antigen (HCVcAg) can be detected in a proportion of individuals. Following the development of the antibody response, HCVcAg becomes complexed with these antibodies specific for HCV.

FIG. 4.5 Approximate Time course of virological and immunological markers of HCV infection with (A) Self-resolving HCV infection, and (B) Chronic HCV infection

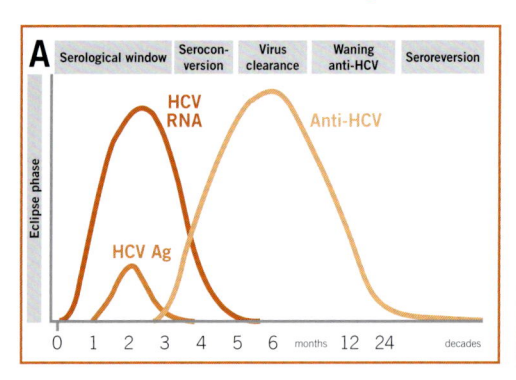

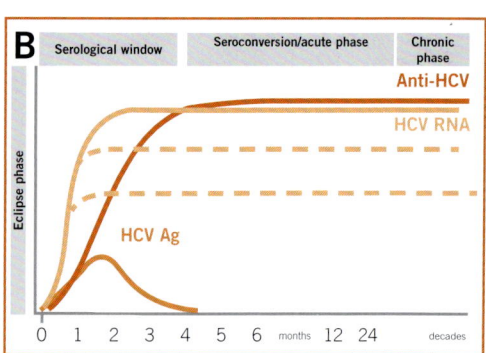

Window period. Assays designed solely to detect antibodies to HCV inevitably have a window period of infectivity in early infection, during which antibodies may be undetectable. This window period can be shortened by utilizing assays that also include direct detection of HCVcAg (50–60 days). HCV RNA is typically not used to determine exposure to HCV, in spite of its short window period (1–2 weeks after the onset of acute infection) primarily because of cost *(135)*. There are increasing reports of occult HCV infection, i.e. HCV RNA detectable in the absence of any serological markers (i.e. HCV seronegative) *(136–138)* which may be due to underlying immunosuppression in, for example, HIV-infected populations.

4.2.5. Prevention of hepatitis C infection

In the absence of a vaccine for hepatitis C, prevention of HCV infection depends upon reducing the risk of exposure to the virus. This is challenging because of the various routes of transmission and the different populations that are affected. Globally, most HCV infections occur in health-care settings as a result of inadequate infection control procedures. WHO has published guidelines with recommendations for preventing health-care-associated HCV infection, and for screening of blood products *(20, 30, 139)*. Universal access to safe blood transfusion requires the implementation of key strategies to ensure access to a safe and sufficient blood supply, including 100% quality-assured testing of donated blood *(139)*. Joint WHO–UNODC guidance recommends a comprehensive package of harm reduction interventions, which comprise nine harm reduction activities specifically for PWID, including the provision of sterile injecting equipment *(140)*, alongside WHO guidance on prevention of viral hepatitis B and C transmission among PWID *(28)*.

4.2.6. Treatment of hepatitis C infection

A new class of medicines, called direct-acting antivirals (DAAs), have transformed the treatment of HCV, with regimens that can be administered for a short duration (as short as eight weeks), resulting in cure rates higher than 90%, but are associated with fewer serious adverse events than the previous interferon-containing regimens. WHO updated its hepatitis C treatment guidelines in 2016 to provide recommendations for the use of new DAAs *(5) (*see *Web annex 3*). There still remains some variation in recommended HCV treatment regimens and duration of therapy by genotype. This requirement to determine a patient's genotype prior to treatment will soon change when antiviral agents that are active against all genotypes (referred to as pangenotypic) are licensed.

5. BACKGROUND – DIAGNOSTICS FOR TESTING FOR HEPATITIS B AND C INFECTION

5.1. Types of viral hepatitis assays

Serological assays are typically used as the first line of the testing strategy to screen for exposure to a virus because of their relatively low cost (compared to NAT), and are therefore used to rule in all individuals who might potentially be infected with HCV or HBV. Serological assays detect the host immune response (antibodies to HCV) or a viral antigen (HBsAg, HCVcAg). They are based on the immunoassay principle, and are available in the form of rapid diagnostic tests (RDTs) or laboratory-based enzyme immunoassays (EIAs), chemoluminescence immunoassays (CLIAs) and electrochemoluminescence immunoassays (ECLs).

In contrast, NAT technologies are typically used to detect the presence of the virus, determine if the infection is active and if the individual would benefit from antiviral treatment. NAT technologies are also used to determine when antiviral treatment should be discontinued (due to non-response or resistance) or to confirm virological cure (HCV) or effective suppression (HBV).

5.2 Serological assays

5.2.1. Rapid diagnostic tests

Rapid diagnostic tests (RDTs) are single-use disposable assays that are provided in simple-to-use formats that generally require no additional reagents except those supplied in the test kit. They are read visually and can give a simple qualitative result in under 30 minutes. Due to their simplicity, cost and rapid turnaround time, they can be performed by trained lay providers or health-care workers, without the need for venepuncture for specimen collection. Quality-assured RDTs are therefore particularly useful in settings where conventional laboratory-based testing services are not available or accessible. They can also be used in outreach programmes (e.g. prison services, prevention and treatment services for people who use drugs).

Most RDTs can be performed with capillary whole blood collected by a finger-stick procedure using a lancet, but many have also been developed for use with venous whole blood, serum or plasma. Certain ones have been validated for use with oral fluid specimens. It is critical to always refer to the manufacturer's instructions for use for specific recommendations on specimen collection. Rapid tests are generally not suitable for testing large numbers of blood samples. The reading of results is dependent on subjective evaluation and no permanent record of the original test results can be kept.

5.2.2. Laboratory-based immunoassays

Most laboratory-based serological immunoassays (EIAs, CLIAs and ECLs) detect antibodies, antigens or a combination of both and differ only in the mode of detection of immune complexes formed. A cut-off value, usually determined by the manufacturer of the assay, specifies the point at which the results are considered to be reactive, and therefore, EIA results are generally reported as optical density divided by the assay cut-off (OD/CO) values. These types of assays are best suited for and most cost–effective to perform in settings with a high throughput of specimens (in excess of 40 per day). They are meant for laboratory- or facility-based testing rather than for use in the community, where infrastructure (electricity, cold storage, climate-controlled rooms) and skilled staff are consistently available, as cold-chain storage of test kits and the use of precision pipettes are usually required. These assays are typically used only with serum or plasma specimens, and therefore require phlebotomy to collect an appropriate specimen.

These assays may be performed either manually or on non-dedicated automated assay or specific dedicated automated systems. Simple immunoanalysers automate a number of the processes and as such require less hands-on time than a manually run EIA. They can therefore be used in range of different situations from high-throughput laboratories for the screening of large numbers of samples with full automation, to medium-sized laboratories with semi-automation, to small laboratories, such as those in remote areas, which conduct a small number of tests manually.

5.2.3. Confirmatory assays

For HBsAg – neutralization assays are used to confirm if observed antigen reactivity is neutralizable upon repeat testing with the same specimen using a neutralization step in the laboratory-based immunoassays, with a specific anti-HBs-containing reagent in the same assay. The result is confirmed when this neutralization reagent can abolish reactivity in the assay in comparison with a control reaction.

For anti-HCV – line immunoassays or immunoblots are serological techniques to confirm the presence of antibodies to HCV that have already been detected by other serological assays. The use of confirmatory assays should be able to provide a definitive result, although these assays are more expensive than other assays and are prone to high rates of indeterminate results. These assays only confirm serostatus and cannot be used to diagnose viraemic active HCV infection.

5.3. Nucleic acid testing technologies

These assays detect the presence of viral nucleic acid – DNA or RNA – through targeting a specific segment of the virus, which is then amplified. The amplification step enables the detection of low levels of the virus in the original specimen, which might not otherwise have been detectable. Laboratory-based technologies for NAT require sophisticated equipment, rigorous laboratory conditions and specimen collection, and highly trained staff who can perform precision steps and avoid contamination. Not all NAT technologies detect all genotypes or subtypes equally well, unless they are optimized to do so. Newly developed NAT technologies that are simpler and more robust are intended for use at or near the point of care, and may avoid some of the logistical and technical disadvantages of laboratory-based NAT technologies.

In addition to NAT assays that target a single virus, multiplex NAT screening assays have been developed, which can detect DNA or RNA from multiple viruses simultaneously.

5.4. Choice of serological assays

Table 5.1 describes the advantages and disadvantages of RDTs and laboratory-based immunoassays. The choice of assay format will depend on a variety of factors, most importantly, performance characteristics (sensitivity and specificity), cost, ease of use and the characteristics of the testing site, such as storage facilities, infrastructure, and level of staff skills. Chapter 15 provides further details on how to set up laboratory services for viral hepatitis testing and selection of an assay, and how to assure the quality of testing.

5.5. Selection of one- or two-assay serological testing strategy

A testing strategy defines the sequence of tests to be followed for a specific testing objective (i.e. to identify infected and non-infected individuals), taking into consideration the anticipated prevalence of HBsAg or HCV antibody in the population(s) to be tested. WHO recommends the use of standardized testing strategies to both maximize the accuracy of HBsAg or HCV antibody testing while simplifying the process through streamlining procurement and training *(11)*. The choice between a one-assay versus two-assay serological testing strategy will depend on the seroprevalence in the population to be tested and diagnostic accuracy (sensitivity and specificity) of the assays used. In these guidelines, we refer to the use of testing strategy only in the context of serological testing and the use of a one- or two-serological assay testing strategy, though it is recognized that other sources refer to the use of a single HCV RNA NAT or core antigen as a one test strategy to replace the need for a two-step process of serological testing followed by NAT.

One-assay serological testing strategy

A one-assay serological testing strategy (Fig. 5.1) is when a single serological test is performed. If the test result is reactive, a "compatible with positive infection" status is reported. If the initial test result is non-reactive, a "negative infection" status is reported. This testing strategy efficiently rules out most uninfected individuals correctly, and rules in those who are likely to be infected and therefore in need of further HBV DNA and HCV RNA NAT testing and staging of liver disease using NITs and clinical evaluation. This testing strategy is particularly suitable for high-prevalence settings due to the relatively higher positive predictive values (PPVs), but needs a highly sensitive and specific assay to maintain acceptable predictive values.

Two-assay serological testing strategy

Two-assay serological testing strategy (Fig. 5.2) differs in that two different assays are used sequentially, to improve the PPV of the testing strategy, and so reduce the number of individuals inappropriately referred on to more specialist services. This can be achieved by either (i) repeating the serological test using a different assay of similar sensitivity, or (ii) in the case of HBsAg, performing a neutralization test using a specific anti-HBs-containing reagent in the same first-line assay after appropriate dilution of the specimen under test.

If the first test result is non-reactive, a "negative infection" status is reported. If both test results are reactive, the status is reported as: "presumptive positive status infection for further diagnostic testing". If the second test result is non-reactive, the status is reported as "infection inconclusive; requires additional testing". If the second assay is less sensitive than the first, then it is likely that some true positives would be discarded if negative on the second test.

Fig. 5.1. One-assay serological testing strategy   **Fig. 5.2.** Two-assay serological testing strategy

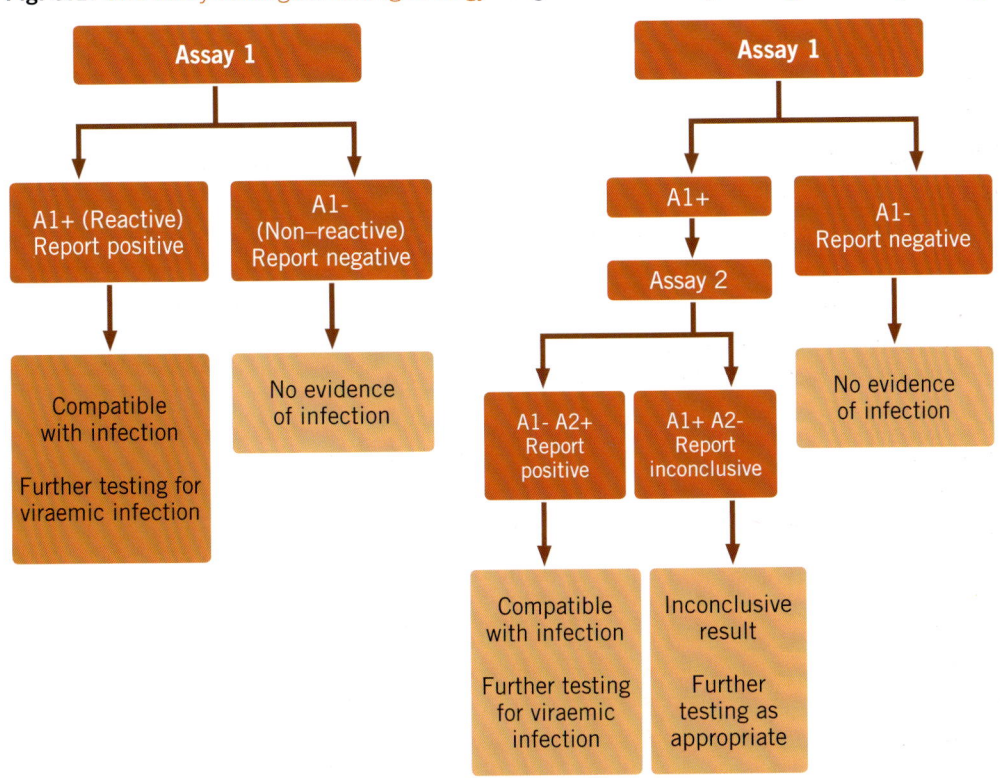

TABLE 5.1 Advantages and disadvantages of different assay formats

Assay	Advantages	Disadvantages
Laboratory-based immunoassays (EIA, CLIA, ECL)	• Currently superior clinical/diagnostic and analytical sensitivity/specificity for HBsAg • High throughput possible (>40 per day per operator) • High throughput greater when using automated immunoanalysers • Objective, automated reading of results, but not for line blots or simple assays • Within-assay procedural quality control	• Requires laboratory facilities, equipment, e.g. EIA plate washers, readers, incubators or immunoanalysers or random-access analysers. • Requires trained laboratory technician • Reagents require refrigeration • Requires venepuncture to obtain specimen • Time to result ~3 hours and generally batched as one run if manual EIA
Rapid diagnostic tests (RDTs)	• Accessible at the lowest level of the health-care system (including community settings) • Does not specifically require laboratory facilities • May be carried out by trained lay providers and health-care workers, as well as laboratory technicians • Can be used with less invasive specimens that do not require venepuncture such as capillary whole blood or oral fluid • If testing at or near to point of care, same-day results are possible, which may reduce number of individuals that are lost to follow up and therefore do not receive their test results • Devices can be stored at 2–30 °C	• Lower clinical and analytical sensitivity/specificity for HBsAg • Less sensitive in certain populations such as immunosuppressed, including HIV-positive individuals • Ineffective within-assay quality control, i.e. most RDTs do not control for specimen addition • Lack of test kit external control reagents for quality control with most RDTs, but some exceptions, e.g. Oraquick • Stability at room temperature is impacted by environmental factors, e.g. heat, humidity, storage conditions • Subjective reading and interpretation of results • Requires manual transcription of testing results into laboratory logbook/testing register, partially mitigated by automated RDT readers
Nucleic acid testing (NAT) technologies	• May be used at or near the point of care • May be carried out by trained lay providers and health-care workers, as well as laboratory technicians • Can be used with less invasive specimens that do not require venepuncture such as capillary whole blood • Devices can be stored at 2–30 °C	• Currently requires laboratory facilities and equipment, but this may not apply to future point-of-care options • Requires trained laboratory technician • Reagents require refrigeration • Requires venepuncture to obtain specimen • Time to result ~3 hours and generally batched as one

PART 2: RECOMMENDATIONS

- **Who to test for HBV and HCV infection**
- **How to test for chronic hepatitis B infection**
  - serology and presence of viraemia
  - monitoring of HBV treatment response
- **How to test for chronic hepatitis C infection**
  - serology and presence of viraemia
  - monitoring of HCV treatment response
- **Use of dried blood spot sampling**
- **Linkage to care and treatment**

6. WHO TO TEST FOR CHRONIC HEPATITIS B OR C INFECTION
– testing approaches and service delivery

6.1. Recommendations

WHO TO TEST FOR CHRONIC HBV INFECTION	
Testing approach and population	**Recommendations***
General population testing	1. In settings with a ≥2% or ≥5%[1] HBsAg seroprevalence in the general population, it is recommended that all adults have routine access to and be offered HBsAg serological testing with linkage to prevention, care and treatment services. General population testing approaches should make use of existing community- or health facility-based testing opportunities or programmes such as at antenatal clinics, HIV or TB clinics. *Conditional recommendation, low quality of evidence*
Routine testing in pregnant women	2. In settings with a ≥2% or ≥5%%[1] HBsAg seroprevalence in the general population, it is recommended that HBsAg serological testing be routinely offered to all pregnant women in antenatal clinics[2], with linkage to prevention, care and treatment services. Couples and partners in antenatal care settings should be offered HBV testing services. *Strong recommendation, low quality of evidence*
Focused testing in most affected populations	3. In all settings (and regardless of whether delivered through facility- or community-based testing), it is recommended that HBsAg serological testing and linkage to care and treatment services be offered to the following individuals: • **Adults and adolescents from populations most affected by HBV infection**[3] (i.e. who are either part of a population with high HBV seroprevalence or who have a history of exposure and/or high-risk behaviours for HBV infection); • **Adults, adolescents and children with a clinical suspicion of chronic viral hepatitis**[4] (i.e. symptoms, signs, laboratory markers); • **Sexual partners, children and other family members, and close household contacts**[5] of those with HBV infection[5]; • **Health-care workers:** in all settings, it is recommended that HBsAg serological testing be offered and hepatitis B vaccination given to all health-care workers who have not been vaccinated previously (*adapted from existing guidance on hepatitis B vaccination*[6]) *Strong recommendation, low quality of evidence*
Blood donors Adapted from existing 2010 WHO guidance (Screening donated blood for transfusion transmissible infections[7])	4. In all settings, screening of blood donors should be mandatory with linkage to care, counselling and treatment for those who test positive.

Abbreviations: HBsAg: hepatitis B surface antigen; PWID: people who inject drugs; MSM: men who have sex with men

*The GRADE system (Grading of Recommendations, Assessment, Development and Evaluation) was used to categorize the strength of recommendations as strong or conditional (based on consideration of the quality of evidence, balance of benefits and harms, acceptability, resource use and programmatic feasibility) and the quality of evidence as high, moderate, low or very low.

[1] A threshold of ≥2% or ≥5% seroprevalence was based on several published thresholds of intermediate or high seroprevalence. The threshold used will depend on other country considerations and epidemiological context.
[2] Many countries have chosen to adopt routine testing in all pregnant women, regardless of seroprevalence in the general population, and particularly where seroprevalence ≥2%. A full vaccination schedule including birth dose should be completed in all infants, in accordance with the WHO position paper on hepatitis B vaccines 2009.[6]
[3] Includes those who are either part of a population with higher seroprevalence (e.g. some mobile/migrant populations from high/intermediate endemic countries, and certain indigenous populations) or who have a history of exposure or high-risk behaviours for HBV infection (e.g. PWID, people in prisons and other closed settings, MSM and sex workers, HIV-infected persons, partners, family members and children of HBV-infected persons).
[4] Features that may indicate underlying chronic HBV infection include clinical evidence of existing liver disease, such as cirrhosis or hepatocellular carcinoma (HCC), or where there is unexplained liver disease, including abnormal liver function tests or liver ultrasound.
[5] In all settings, it is recommended that HBsAg serological testing with hepatitis B vaccination of those who are HBsAg negative and not previously vaccinated be offered to all children with parents or siblings diagnosed with HBV infection or with clinical suspicion of hepatitis, through community- or facility-based testing.
[6] WHO position paper. Hepatitis B vaccines. Wkly Epidemiol Rec. 2009;4 (84):405–20.
[7] Screening donated blood for transfusion transmissible infections. Geneva: World Health Organization; 2010.

WHO TO TEST FOR CHRONIC HCV INFECTION	
Testing approach and population	**Recommendations***
Focused testing in most affected populations	1. In all settings (and regardless of whether delivered through facility- or community-based testing), it is recommended that serological testing for HCV antibody (anti-HCV)[1] be offered with linkage to prevention, care and treatment services to the following individuals: • **Adults and adolescents from populations most affected by HCV infection**[2] (i.e. who are either part of a population with high HCV seroprevalence or who have a history of exposure and/or high-risk behaviours for HCV infection); • **Adults, adolescents and children with a clinical suspicion of chronic viral hepatitis**[3] (i.e. symptoms, signs, laboratory markers). *Strong recommendation, low quality of evidence* *Note: Periodic re-testing using HCV NAT should be considered for those with ongoing risk of acquisition or reinfection.*
General population testing	2. In settings with a ≥2% or ≥5%[4] HCV antibody seroprevalence in the general population, it is recommended that all adults have access to and be offered HCV serological testing with linkage to prevention, care and treatment services. General population testing approaches should make use of existing community- or facility-based testing opportunities or programmes such as HIV or TB clinics, drug treatment services and antenatal clinics[5]. *Conditional recommendation, low quality of evidence*
Birth cohort testing	3. This approach may be applied to specific identified birth cohorts of older persons at higher risk of infection[6] and morbidity within populations that have an overall lower general prevalence. *Conditional recommendation, low quality of evidence*

Abbreviations: NAT: nucleic acid test; anti-HCV: HCV antibody; PWID: people who inject drugs; MSM: men who have sex with men

*The GRADE system (Grading of Recommendations, Assessment, Development and Evaluation) was used to categorize the strength of recommendations as strong or conditional (based on consideration of the quality of evidence, balance of benefits and harms, acceptability, resource use and programmatic feasibility) and the quality of evidence as high, moderate, low or very low.

[1] This may include fourth-generation combined antibody/antigen assays

[2] Includes those who are either part of a population with higher seroprevalence (e.g. some mobile/migrant populations from high/intermediate endemic countries, and certain indigenous populations) or who have a history of exposure or high-risk behaviours for HCV infection (e.g. PWID, people in prisons and other closed settings, MSM and sex workers, and HIV-infected persons, children of mothers with chronic HCV infection especially if HIV-coinfected).

[3] Features that may indicate underlying chronic HCV infection include clinical evidence of existing liver disease, such as cirrhosis or hepatocellular carcinoma (HCC), or where there is unexplained liver disease, including abnormal liver function tests or liver ultrasound.

[4] A threshold of ≥2% or ≥5% seroprevalence was based on several published thresholds of intermediate and high seroprevalence. The threshold used will depend on other country considerations and epidemiological context.

[5] Routine testing of pregnant women for HCV infection is currently not recommended.

[6] Because of historical exposure to unscreened or inadequately screened blood products and/or poor injection safety.

6.2. Background

Viral hepatitis testing can be delivered to different populations and in different settings as part of **general population testing**, and/or a **focused testing approach in most affected or high-risk populations**, delivered through either **health facility-based or community-based testing**. Chapter 17 provides additional details on the different facility- and community-based testing approaches available. Chapter 18 provides additional guidance on testing in specific populations.

Different hepatitis testing approaches

There are several possible approaches to testing for HBV and HCV infection.

1. **General population testing.** This approach refers to routine testing throughout the entire population without attempting to identify high-risk behaviours or characteristics. It means that all members of the population should have potential access to the testing services. This approach might be indicated for those countries with an intermediate or high HBV or HCV seroprevalence. At present, only Japan recommends HCV testing for all individuals once in their lives regardless of demographics or specific behavioural risk.

2. **Focused or targeted testing of specific high-risk groups.** This approach refers to testing of specific populations who are most affected by hepatitis B or C infection, either because they are part of a population with high HBV or HCV seroprevalence (such as some migrant populations and some indigenous populations), or have a high risk of acquisition because of risk behaviours and/or exposures. This includes PWID, people in prisons and other closed settings, MSM and sex workers, HIV-infected persons, partners or family members of infected persons, and health-care workers. It may also involve testing on the basis of clinical suspicion of viral hepatitis (i.e. symptoms, signs or abnormal liver function tests or ultrasound scan).

3. **Routine antenatal clinic (ANC) testing.** This means routine testing of pregnant women especially in settings where there is an intermediate or high seroprevalence, to identify women in need of antiviral treatment for their own health and additional interventions to reduce MTCT of viral hepatitis.

4. **"Birth cohort" testing.** This approach means routine testing among easily identified age or demographic groups (i.e. specific "birth cohorts") known to have high HCV prevalence due to past generalized exposures that have since been identified and removed. General one-time screening among this population avoids the need to identify risk behaviour. Most countries have at least some component of a "birth cohort" epidemic profile for HCV. Use of a birth cohort approach to HCV testing is currently recommended only in the United States.

5. **Blood donor screening.** WHO already recommends universal blood donor screening for viral hepatitis in order to prevent transmission of bloodborne viruses to the recipient

(20). However, at present, this is rarely accompanied by the HBsAg- or HCV antibody-positive donors being informed of this positive result, counselled and linked to care for clinical evaluation and treatment *(141)*.

Service delivery of testing approaches (health facility- or community-based)

The testing approaches described above can be offered and delivered using both health-facility and/or community-based testing services.

Health-facility-based testing includes primary care clinics, inpatient wards and outpatient clinics, including specialist dedicated clinics such as HIV, STI and TB clinics, in district and provincial or regional hospitals as well as their laboratories, and in private clinical services.

Community-based testing can be offered and delivered using outreach (mobile) approaches in general and key populations; home-based testing (or door-to-door outreach); testing in workplaces, places of worship, parks, bars and other venues; in schools and other educational establishments; as well as through campaigns (e.g. screening for HIV or malaria alongside that for noncommunicable diseases such as diabetes and hypertension). Although many of these approaches were developed to increase the coverage and impact of HIV testing *(11)*, they are equally applicable to the delivery of hepatitis testing.

6A TESTING APPROACHES TO DETECT CHRONIC HEPATITIS B

6.3. Summary of the evidence

The evidence base for different HBV testing approaches (general population or focused testing) remains very limited, especially in LMICs, and relies largely on observational data and modelling. Although there are descriptive data showing that focused testing can increase the uptake of HBV testing, and detection rate of CHB cases, data showing impact on patient-important outcomes are limited *(142)*. There is also a lack of evidence on and uncertainty regarding how successful focused testing is in reaching specific populations. For these reasons, a formal systematic review of the impact and cost–effectiveness of different testing approaches was precluded, and an updated narrative review of evidence was undertaken. The overall quality of evidence was therefore rated as low.

There were 32 published studies of which nine studies met the inclusion criteria – all but one study were from HICs with low HBV prevalence (see *Web annex 5.1*). Two studies evaluated the cost–effectiveness of offering testing and treatment to the general population (one from the United States *(143)* and the other from west Africa *(144)*), and seven studies had examined targeted risk-group testing in migrant populations *(145–150)* or "high-risk" groups *(151)*. Several studies were based on modelling simulations using hypothetical data. Various outcome measures were used, including cost per quality-adjusted life-year (QALY) gained, cost per life-year (LY) saved and cost per case tested.

General population testing. The two studies performed in the United States and West Africa showed that offering HBsAg testing to the general population with provision of antiviral treatment in those eligible is cost–effective in both high-income *(143)* and low-income settings *(144)*, even down to a population prevalence as low as 0.3% and 1.5%, respectively. In addition, the feasibility of large-scale testing and treatment in sub-Saharan Africa based on real-world cost and effectiveness data was demonstrated by the PROLIFICA (Prevention of Liver Fibrosis and Liver Cancer in Africa) study in west Africa *(152)*. This study screened almost 10 000 adults for HBsAg using an active outreach method at the community level in the Gambia and Senegal, followed by full clinical assessment of those found HBsAg positive, and provision of antiviral treatment if they met eligibility criteria. They showed this community-based screen-and-treat strategy was cost-effective compared to the status quo.

Focused risk-based testing. Testing and treatment of migrant or refugee populations in HICs was also found to be a cost-effective intervention in seven studies from Canada, the United States and Europe *(145–150)*.

Pregnant women. Although the cost–effectiveness of HBsAg testing of pregnant women in ANC to reduce MTCT and benefits to the child has been addressed in several studies, there were none identified that considered interventions and antiviral treatment for the benefit of the mother to reduce her risk of progression of liver disease.

Drivers of cost–effectiveness. These analyses identified several key drivers of cost–effectiveness for countries to consider when planning testing approaches. These include: (i) **Drug and testing costs.** The key driver of the cost–effectiveness of a test-and-treat strategy reported is the cost of the antiviral drug *(144, 146, 147)*, and to a lesser extent testing costs *(145, 147)*. In the PROLIFICA study, despite an active community-based screening campaign, testing costs were low (US$ 7.43 per person offered screening) and the intervention remained cost-effective even if there was a threefold increase in testing costs *(144)*. (ii) **Linkage to care and adherence.** Adherence to treatment and linkage to care were reported as key drivers of cost–effectiveness in several studies *(148)*, but not in the PROLIFICA study *(152)*. (iii) **Uptake of testing** was not identified as a key driver of incremental cost-effectiveness ratio (ICER) in any of the studies. However, this does not imply that high participation levels in screening are not important. The implication of this result is that it is likely to be worthwhile performing screening and providing treatment, even if participation in screening may be low, in part because testing costs are low relative to the costs and health benefits of treatment for those who are infected. HBsAg prevalence also had a relatively small influence on cost–effectiveness across a wide range of prevalence levels examined.

6.4. Rationale for the recommendations on testing approaches for HBV infection

In developing recommendations on which populations to test and what testing approaches to use, the Guidelines Development Group first considered the primary goals of testing *(153)*: (i) to identify those in greatest need of treatment to reduce morbidity and mortality from HBV-related chronic liver disease; (ii) to reduce the risk of acquisition of disease, by vaccinating those who do not have HBV infection but remain at risk; and (iii) to reduce the risk of mother-to-child vertical transmission and so have benefits that extend beyond the person tested to others. These considerations were then balanced with the need for recommendations that are feasible and implementable by health programmes in LMICs.

Overall, there was a very limited evidence base for the impact of different testing approaches (general population or focused high-risk) as well as for different settings (community- versus health facility-based). Therefore, recommendations were formulated based on consideration of evidence mainly from cost–effectiveness analyses together with data on HBsAg seroprevalence in different settings and populations, and in the general population with considerations of feasibility and cost. The caveats of extrapolating cost-effectiveness data from HICs to LMICs were recognized. The Guidelines Development Group recommended the use of three key testing approaches: **routine testing in the general population; focused testing in most affected populations** because of higher-risk behaviours or exposures; and **routine ANC testing.** These can be implemented both in health-care facilities and in the community, as appropriate to the local epidemiology and context.

Balance of benefits and harms

General population testing. In settings where there is an HBsAg prevalence ≥2% in the general population, focused testing in higher-risk populations alone will be insufficient to identify many of those infected and in need of treatment. Additional general population testing approaches that use community- as well as health facility-based testing programmes are therefore needed to increase the coverage and impact of HBV testing. Although general population testing was estimated to be cost–effective down to prevalence levels <1%, the Guidelines Development Group proposed a higher threshold of ≥2% to reflect the well-accepted thresholds for defining intermediate (≥2%)/high (≥5%) seroprevalence *(154)*. The Guidelines Development Group recognized that the threshold used by countries will depend on other country considerations and epidemiological context. For this reason, a conditional recommendation was made.

Focused risk-based testing in populations with high-risk behaviour or exposure to HBV infection. Certain populations are well recognized to be at high risk of acquisition and transmission of HBV infection (Table 4.1), and therefore should be prioritized for testing in all epidemic settings. These include people living with HIV, PWID, MSM, sex workers, people in prisons and other closed settings, some mobile/migrant populations from high/intermediate-endemic countries, some indigenous populations, children born to HBsAg-positive mothers, especially if they did not receive timely infant vaccination, and other family members, sexual partners and close household contacts of those with HBV infection; and health-care workers. In high-endemic settings, a clinically guided testing approach among adults and children with a clinical suspicion of chronic viral hepatitis (i.e. clinical symptoms or signs, or abnormal liver function tests or ultrasound scan) will identify a larger proportion of infected persons.

Key benefits of focused testing

1. Focused testing in health facilities can successfully increase the uptake of viral hepatitis testing, case detection rate, and referrals to specialist-level care and other important services.

2. Focused testing approaches can use existing opportunities and infrastructure for health facility-based testing (HIV, STI, and TB outpatient clinics, drug treatment programmes, primary care settings, inpatient and outpatient settings), as well as community-based testing.

3. Focused testing of high-prevalence populations or of those in settings where there is a large proportion of such persons (e.g. harm reduction and drug treatment services for PWID) or a clinically guided approach based on clinical suspicion is likely to be associated with higher rates of case–finding. This approach will generally be cost–effective compared to generalized testing, especially in low- and concentrated-epidemic settings.

4. It is recognized that many high HBV-prevalence countries currently lack the resources to undertake general population screening, and therefore focused risk-based testing may be more readily feasible and cost–effective, particularly if it makes use of existing health-facility infrastructure and staff.

Despite the limited formal evaluation of focused testing in high-risk groups and low quality of evidence, a strong recommendation was made because of the overall benefits of focused testing approaches.

Pregnant women – routine testing in antenatal clinics. The Guidelines Development Group strongly recommended routine HBsAg testing in ANC, despite limited or low-quality evidence, for several reasons.

1. To benefit their offspring through interventions to significantly reduce MTCT of HBV infection *(6)*. This is because in high-prevalence, resource-limited settings, HBV is mainly transmitted through MTCT and early childhood horizontal transmissions. Infants born to HBV-infected mothers are at high risk for both acquisition of HBV infection and development of chronic infection (90%). Therefore, key interventions in this group could significantly reduce the burden of disease in the long term.

2. To enable women to have knowledge of their HBV serostatus (together with their offspring and partners), allowing them to benefit for their own health through linkage to assessment and treatment services.

3. Although a systematic review of cost–effectiveness studies on routine antenatal testing in LMICs was not undertaken, this would likely be cost-effective, since testing of mothers for HBV infection has benefits for both the child (reduced transmission) and mother (reduced morbidity).

4. There is already universal HIV testing in ANC which has proved feasible and acceptable in many countries *(6, 11, 153)*, and addition of HBV testing would be relatively low cost. Although many countries recommend routine screening of women for HBV infection in ANC, the proportion who are screened in many LMICs remains low *(157)*.

Couples and partner testing in ANC. HIV testing of the partners of women attending ANC is now a focus in 21 priority countries aiming for elimination of MTCT (eMTCT) of HIV. Since these countries are also all highly endemic for HBV, this provides a unique opportunity to integrate concurrent HBV testing for partners of women with CHB, or chronic HCV infection if risk factors are present, despite the lack of specific evidence for couples and partner testing for hepatitis in ANC.

Blood donor screening. WHO already recommends blood donor screening for HBV, HCV, HIV and syphilis in order to prevent transmission of bloodborne viruses to the recipient *(20)*. However, this is rarely accompanied by the HBsAg or HCV antibody positive donor being informed of this positive result, counselled and linked into care for clinical evaluation and treatment *(141)*. As part of the PROLIFICA study in west Africa, in addition to HBsAg testing and treatment in the community, blood donors who had tested HBsAg positive at the blood bank were linked to specialist care *(152)*. A higher proportion of blood donors were HBsAg positive and requiring treatment, but had a lower rate of linkage to care. Although a formal cost–effectiveness analysis was not done, these factors are likely to make testing, linkage and treatment of blood donors even more cost-effective compared to community-based testing. However, as blood donors constitute only a small fraction of the population, this strategy is likely to be limited in its reach and population-level effectiveness, and probably should be seen as a complementary, rather than an alternative to a wider screening strategy.

Acceptability, values and preferences

A values and preferences survey of 104 stakeholders from 43 (20 high-income, 23 low- and middle-income) countries provided additional strong support for testing of specific populations: blood donors (>85%), children born to HBV-infected mothers (75%), persons living with HIV (65%), pregnant women (78%), MSM (45%), sex workers (45%), prisoners (25%) and those chronically ill (around 25%). General population testing for HBV infection was supported by only one third of respondents.

6B TESTING APPROACHES TO DETECT CHRONIC HEPATITIS C

6.5. Summary of the evidence

A systematic review and meta-analysis of the impact and cost–effectiveness of different HCV testing approaches (general population or focused testing) was precluded by the limited number of available studies and because of the heterogeneity of settings and populations studied and outcomes measured. Therefore, a narrative review was undertaken in different settings, alongside consideration of recent systematic reviews of HCV seroprevalence in different populations. The three main testing approaches evaluated were (i) routine testing throughout the entire population; (ii) focused or targeted testing of the highest-risk groups; and (iii) routine testing among specific birth cohorts. The overall quality of evidence was rated as low.

Overall, there were 31 relevant studies based on a previously published systematic review *(158)* and 12 additional studies identified in an updated search *(159–192)* (*see Web annex 5.2*). The majority of studies were from Europe or the US, and very few from LMICs. Fourteen studies evaluated testing in the general population *(125, 159–171)*; 13 in PWID and STD clinics *(174–177, 179–181)*; three in recipients of blood transfusions *(160, 161, 182)*; one among HIV-infected MSM *(183)*; two among pregnant women *(184, 185)*, and two in other populations *(186, 187)*.

Focused testing. Focused testing of PWID, people in prisons or closed settings and HIV-infected MSM was shown to be cost-effective in all settings *(159, 176, 180, 183, 188)*. This was the case among PWID even when the studies assumed poor follow-up rates, limited access to therapy *(159, 180)* and a high risk of reinfection. The higher the treatment rates, the greater the population impact, and the more cost–effective HCV case-finding becomes *(189)*. Among prisoners, targeting testing to those prisoners with a history of injection drug use further improved cost–effectiveness *(176)*. Among HIV-positive MSM population *(183)*, cost–effectiveness was dependent on appropriate linkage to effective therapy and retention in care.

"Birth-cohort" testing. Most countries have at least some component of a "birth cohort" HCV epidemic (i.e. of easily identified age or demographic groups known to have a higher HCV prevalence), and several cost–effectiveness studies from the US and Portugal show that birth cohort testing is cost effective when compared to risk-based screening or current testing approaches *(125, 166, 168, 190)*.

Routine testing in the general population. A major limitation of existing cost–effectiveness studies of testing in the general population is that they were conducted based on the use of interferon-based regimens and not using the new

DAA curative treatments, and in HICs *(125, 151, 160, 162, 163, 165, 167, 169, 170)*. Only one cost–effectiveness study has been undertaken in a LMIC – in Egypt, which has a very high prevalence of disease. Routine testing was shown to be cost-effective even when treatment was based on use of pegylated interferon (PEG-IFN) and ribavirin (PEG-RBV) *(191)*.

Drivers of cost–effectiveness. In all analyses, the cost–effectiveness of testing for HCV was most sensitive to variations in prevalence, treatment efficacy (i.e. the replacement of IFN/RBV with significantly improved efficacy of DAAs), progression rates from chronic HCV to cirrhosis, and levels of linkage to care and treatment *(164, 165, 170)*. It was relatively insensitive to costs of screening and treatment.

Based on this narrative review of heterogeneous studies of cost–effectiveness of testing approaches from HICs, the overall quality of evidence was rated as low.

6.6. Rationale for the recommendations on testing approaches for HCV infection

The Guidelines Development Group recognized that HCV epidemics around the world are heterogeneous but are largely represented by mixtures of three main epidemic patterns for which a specific testing approach is appropriate. These are as follows:

1. **Infection related to high-risk behaviours** – requiring focused or targeted testing in the highest-risk groups;

2. **Infection related to past generalized exposures that have since been identified and removed (i.e. "birth cohort epidemic")** – requiring routine testing among specific birth cohorts that are readily identified and that have a high prevalence of HCV infection;

3. **Generalized population epidemic with high prevalence** generally related to a widespread, often iatrogenic, exposure – requiring routine testing throughout the entire population.

Few countries have epidemics that fall into one of the above three profiles. Rather, the majority have mixed epidemic profiles, with some combination of all these components. Determining the optimal strategic mix of HCV testing approaches to increase the diagnosis rate, and in particular, the approach to testing outside of high-risk risk groups will depend on a country's unique HCV epidemic profile (*see* chapter 19).

The lack of evidence from LMICs on evaluation of different testing approaches was noted. Testing in high-risk behaviour groups and in settings with a large proportion of patients such as PWID, MSM, prisoners, HIV-infected persons and commercial sex workers was cost–effective in all settings. The best approach to testing outside of high-risk risk groups depends on a country's unique HCV epidemiology. Most countries have at least some component of a "birth cohort" epidemic, and "birth cohort" testing is likely to be cost–effective in most settings. In most epidemic settings, routine screening of the entire population may not be cost–effective.

Balance of benefits and harms

Focused risk-based testing. The Guidelines Development Group considered that those specific populations at the highest risk of acquisition and transmission of HCV such as PWID, people in prisons and other closed settings, MSM and sex workers should be prioritized for testing, as this was both cost–effective and had a high yield of case-finding. In settings with a high prevalence, this also means focused testing of adults and children with a clinical suspicion of chronic viral hepatitis infection (i.e. clinical symptoms or signs of cirrhosis or HCC, or abnormal liver function tests or ultrasound scan). Other higher-risk groups for focused testing include persons who have had tattoos, body piercing or scarification, unsafe medical procedures, received blood products in countries where screening of blood is not carried out routinely, as well as partners and close contacts of people with HCV infection. The Guidelines Development Group recognized that the priority groups will differ across countries and settings, and that it will be important to ensure adequate linkage to care after diagnosis.

Children. The Guidelines Development Group also considered that screening was indicated for children born to mothers with HCV infection (especially if also HIV infected) because of an increased risk for MTCT after 18 months of age.

Key benefits of focused testing

1. Focused testing in health facilities can successfully increase the uptake of viral hepatitis testing, case detection rate, and referral to specialist-level care and other key services.

2. Focused testing of these populations can be offered in high-prevalence settings such as harm reduction and drug treatment services for PWID. Other existing opportunities for health-facility -based testing can also be used (e.g. dedicated HIV, STI and TB outpatient clinics, and other primary care, outpatient and inpatient settings), as well as testing in the community.

3. A clinically guided testing approach is also likely to identify a larger proportion of people with HCV in highly endemic settings and therefore result in a lower cost per positive person found.

Risks of focused testing. Although ascertaining high-risk behaviours is a very effective way of identifying persons for testing, many people are unwilling to admit to stigmatizing behaviours, and health-care providers are also reluctant to ask (or have too limited time). As a result, medical records capture this information poorly, as the use of electronic medical records to flag high-risk persons for testing is limited.

Birth-cohort testing. The best approach to testing outside of groups with high risk behaviour or exposure depends on a country's unique HCV epidemiology. For example, in many settings, unsafe injection practices will probably have more of an impact on HCV prevalence than illicit injecting drug use. The Guidelines Development Group concluded that whenever there is an easily identified demographic group that has a high HCV prevalence (e.g. all individuals born in a certain time period), routine testing for HCV within that cohort, i.e. "birth cohort" testing will likely be cost–effective and should be considered. This will largely apply to those countries where routine screening of the blood supply for HCV in the 1990s and improvements in injection safety practices have since removed the exposure risk. A conditional recommendation was made mainly because of low quality of evidence.

Key benefits of birth cohort testing

1. Recent studies in the US showed birth cohort screening to be cost–effective when compared with risk-based screening. While typically identified as being the infection pattern in North America and Europe, many countries have at least some component of "birth cohort" epidemic in their HCV epidemiology, and therefore "birth cohort" testing is likely to be cost–effective in most settings.

2. A key advantage of this generally one-off screening approach is that it avoids the need to identify specific behavioural risks as the basis for screening, because providers may not be skilled at identifying high-risk behaviours, and individuals may not remember that they received a blood product, or report to previous risk-taking behaviour on direct questioning.

Key risks of birth cohort testing. More recent data suggest that a significant proportion of the HCV-infected population is not captured as part of birth cohort screening *(192)*. A further challenge is that this approach requires reliable data on both the age distribution of the population and prevalence according to age, which is not available in most countries.

General population testing. Routine screening for HCV in the general population was generally not considered cost–effective outside specific settings with high general population prevalence. The application of a one-off birth cohort screening approach to testing the general population will be more widely applicable. Therefore, a conditional recommendation was made to support consideration of general population testing in intermediate- and high-prevalence settings.

Acceptability, values and preferences

A values and preferences survey of 104 stakeholders from 43 (20 high-income, 23 low- and middle-income) countries identified the following target populations as priority for hepatitis C testing: blood donors (>85%), children born to HCV-infected mothers (55%), persons living with HIV (50%), pregnant women (40%), MSM (25%), prisoners (25%), sex workers (<10%), and those chronically ill (25%). General population testing for HCV infection was supported by 30% of respondents.

6C SERVICE DELIVERY OF HEPATITIS B AND C TESTING

The Guidelines Development Group recommended the use of various health facility or community-based testing opportunities in the general population or focused on high-risk groups because of the overall benefits of these testing approaches. However, this was conditional because of the currently limited evidence base. Chapter 17 provides specific examples of the many different types of facility and community-based testing approaches.

6.7 Rationale for the recommendations on community-based testing

Balance of benefits and harms

Strategies for the delivery of general population or focused testing approaches include door-to-door/home-based testing and mobile outreach campaigns, and testing in workplaces, parks, bars, places of worship and educational establishments.

Benefits of community-based testing

1. There is some evidence that the offer of HBsAg testing in community settings may increase the acceptance and uptake of testing, and rates of early diagnosis *(193)*.

2. The benefits of **community-based testing** to access the general population are that it can also reach first-time testers and people who seldom use clinical services or are unlikely to go to a facility. This particularly includes those from key and vulnerable populations in all settings *(11, 194)*, but also those who are asymptomatic.

3. Community-based focused testing of high-risk groups. Innovative models of care have been developed and effectively implemented in many settings to provide integrated HIV *(194)* and hepatitis testing, and opioid substitution therapy (OST) services for PWID in community drug treatment services. Many of these programmes provide additional interventions, including education, harm reduction, mental health services, other general medical services, and referrals to care and treatment *(195)*. These models can provide a framework for lower-income countries to expand viral hepatitis testing and treatment for at-risk populations.

Risks of community-based testing. Key challenges encountered in delivering community-based HIV testing include ensuring the availability and accessibility of prevention, care and treatment services; and risks associated with potential lack of confidentiality in these settings, and associated stigmatization and discrimination. These will need to be addressed while delivering community-based hepatitis testing.

7. HOW TO TEST FOR CHRONIC HEPATITIS B INFECTION – choice of serological assay and testing strategy

7.1. Recommendations

HOW TO TEST FOR CHRONIC HBV INFECTION AND MONITOR TREATMENT RESPONSE	
Topic	**Recommendations**

Which serological assays to use	• For the diagnosis of chronic HBV infection in adults, adolescents and children (>12 months of age[1]), a serological assay (in either RDT or laboratory-based immunoassay format[2]) that meets minimum quality, safety and performance standards[3] (*with regard to both analytical and clinical sensitivity and specificity*) is recommended to detect hepatitis B surface antigen (HBsAg).
	   - In settings where existing laboratory testing is already available and accessible, laboratory-based immunoassays are recommended as the preferred assay format.
	   - In settings where there is limited access to laboratory testing and/or in populations where access to rapid testing would facilitate linkage to care and treatment, use of RDTs is recommended to improve access.
	Strong recommendation, low/moderate quality of evidence

Serological testing strategies	• In settings or populations with an HBsAg seroprevalence of ≥0.4%[4], a single serological assay for detection of HBsAg is recommended, prior to further evaluation for HBV DNA and staging of liver disease. • In settings or populations with a low HBsAg seroprevalence of <0.4%[4], confirmation of HBsAg positivity on the same immunoassay with a neutralization step or a second different RDT assay for detection of HBsAg may be considered[5]. *Conditional recommendation, low quality of evidence*

Abbreviations: ALT: alanine aminotransferase; AST: aspartate aminotransferase; APRI: aspartate-to-platelet ratio index; HBeAg: HBV e antigen; HBsAg: HBV surface antigen; NAT: nucleic acid test; RDT: rapid diagnostic test

[1] A full vaccination schedule including birth dose should be completed in all infants in accordance with the WHO position paper on Hepatitis B vaccines, 2009. Testing of exposed infants is problematic within the first six months of life as HBsAg and hepatitis B DNA may be inconsistently detectable in infected infants. Exposed infants should be tested for HBsAg between 6 and 12 months of age to screen for evidence of hepatitis B infection. In all age groups, acute HBV infection can be confirmed by the presence of HBsAg and IgM anti-HBc. CHB is diagnosed if there is persistence of HBsAg for six months or more.

[2] Laboratory-based immunoassays include enzyme immunoassay (EIA), chemoluminescence immunoassay (CLIA), and electrochemoluminescence assay (ECL).

[3] Assays should meet minimum acceptance criteria of either WHO prequalification of in vitro diagnostics (IVDs) or a stringent regulatory review for IVDs. All IVDs should be used in accordance with manufacturers' instructions for use and where possible at testing sites enrolled in a national or international external quality assessment scheme.

[4] Based on results of predictive modelling of positive predictive values according to different thresholds of seroprevalence in populations to be tested, and assay diagnostic performance.

[5] A repeat HBsAg assay after 6 months is also a common approach used to confirm chronicity of HBV infection.

FIG. 7.1 WHO-recommended testing strategies for diagnosis of chronic HBV infection with (A) Single assay with HBsAg seroprevalence above 0.4%, and (B) Two assays with HBsAg seroprevalence below 0.4%

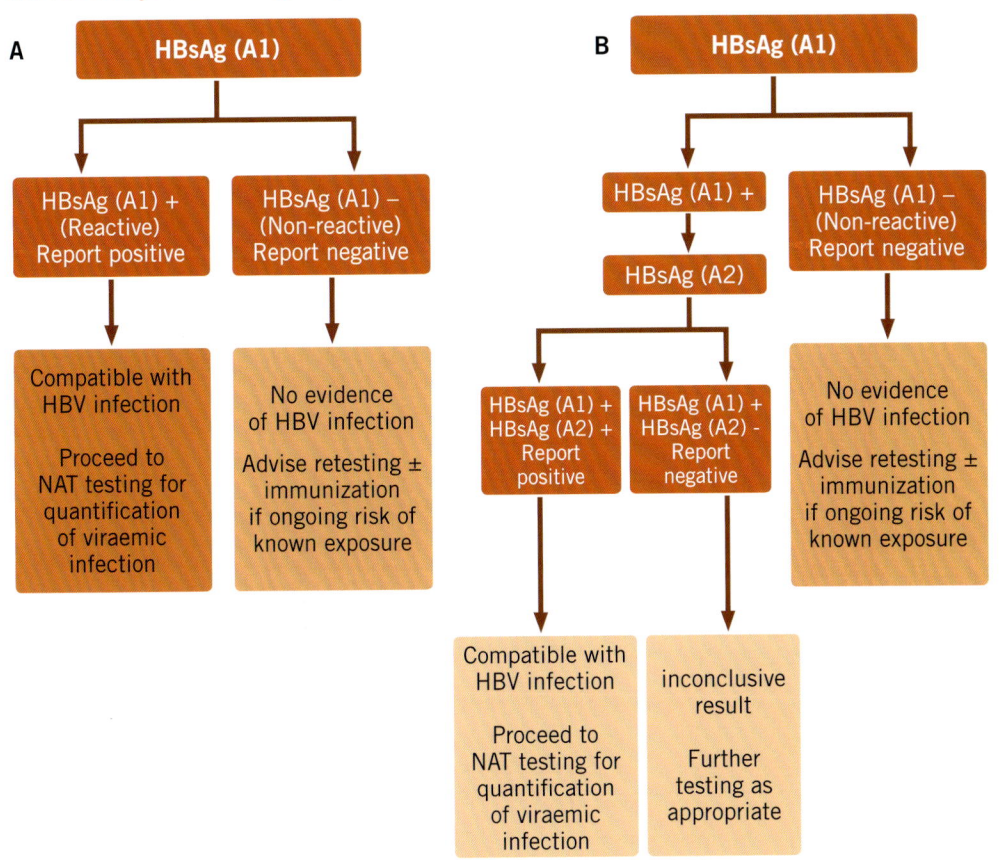

A

HBsAg (A1)
├── HBsAg (A1) + (Reactive) Report positive → Compatible with HBV infection. Proceed to NAT testing for quantification of viraemic infection
└── HBsAg (A1) − (Non-reactive) Report negative → No evidence of HBV infection. Advise retesting ± immunization if ongoing risk of known exposure

B

HBsAg (A1)
├── HBsAg (A1) + → HBsAg (A2)
│   ├── HBsAg (A1) + HBsAg (A2) + Report positive → Compatible with HBV infection. Proceed to NAT testing for quantification of viraemic infection
│   └── HBsAg (A1) + HBsAg (A2) − Report negative → inconclusive result. Further testing as appropriate
└── HBsAg (A1) − (Non-reactive) Report negative → No evidence of HBV infection. Advise retesting ± immunization if ongoing risk of known exposure

7.2. Background

Testing to determine chronic HBV infection is conducted using serological assays, either RDTs or EIAs that detect HBsAg. Confirmation of the presence of HBsAg may be carried out by performing either a neutralization step in the same assay, or by repeating HBsAg testing using a different assay of similar sensitivity (i.e. two-assay serological testing strategy). The choice of which format of serological assays to use will depend on a variety of factors, such as the performance criteria of the test (sensitivity and specificity), cost, ease of use and the characteristics of the testing site, such as storage facilities, infrastructure, and level of staff skills. Chapter 5 provides a background to different IVDs and Table 5.1, summarizes the advantages and disadvantages of laboratory-based immunoassays and RDTs.

WHO recommends the use of standardized testing strategies both to maximize the accuracy of HBsAg testing while minimizing cost and simplifying the process. **A testing strategy** describes a testing sequence for a specific testing objective, taking into consideration the anticipated prevalence of HBsAg in the population. *See* section 5.1.6 for a background on one- and two-assay serological testing strategies. The choice between a one- versus two-assay serological testing strategy will depend on the HBsAg prevalence in the population as well as diagnostic accuracy (sensitivity and specificity) of the HBsAg assays used.

A one-assay serological testing strategy (Fig. 7.1A) is when a single serological test is performed. If the test result is reactive, a "compatible with HBsAg-positive" status is reported. If the initial test result is non-reactive, an "HBsAg-negative" status is reported. The addition of a second serological test with **a two-assay serological testing strategy (Fig. 7.1B)** will generally improve the PPV (i.e. the proportion of individuals detected that actually have HBV infection), reduce the number of false-positive results and therefore the number of individuals inappropriately referred on to specialist services.

7.3. Summary of the evidence
Which serological assay to use

A systematic review (see *Web annex 5.3*) compared the diagnostic performance (sensitivity, specificity, positive and negative predictive values) of commercially available serological assays (RDTs and EIAs[1]) for the detection of HBsAg, when compared to a laboratory-based immunoassay reference standard (with or without a neutralization step). The review identified 30 studies *(197–226)* from 23 countries with varying prevalence of hepatitis B and evaluated 33 different RDTs. There were five studies of eight different EIAs against an immunoassay reference standard *(214, 223, 227–229)*. A mixture of serum, plasma, capillary and venous whole blood specimens were used for RDTs, but only serum or plasma was used for EIAs. Seven studies assessed performance using capillary or venous whole blood *(202, 206, 210, 215, 216, 218, 226)*. Sample size varied from 25 to 3928, and populations studied included healthy volunteers and blood donors, at-risk populations, pregnant women, incarcerated adults, and patients with confirmed hepatitis B.

RDTs. In 30 studies *(197–226)* of 33 different RDTs, the pooled clinical sensitivity of RDTs against different EIA reference standards was 90.0% (95% CI: 89.1–90.8) and pooled specificity was 99.5% (95% CI: 99.4–99.5) (Table 7.1).
Brands: there was significant variation in performance between RDT brands and within the same brand of RDT, with sensitivity ranging from 50% to 100% and specificity from 69% to 100%.
Specimen type: results for capillary whole blood specimens were comparable to serum but less heterogeneous.

---
[1] CLIAs and ECLs were not included specifically in the research question. It is acknowledged that high-income settings are likely to be using these formats of immunoassays.

EIAs. In five studies *(214, 223, 227–229)* of eight EIAs there was wide variation in EIA performance, with sensitivity ranging from 74% to 100% and specificity from 88% to 100%. The pooled sensitivity was 88.9% (95% CI: 87–90.6) and pooled specificity was 98.4% (95% CI: 97.8–98.8).

RDTs and EIAs in HIV-positive persons. Five studies *(212, 214, 215, 218, 222)* evaluated three different RDTs against different EIA reference standards. The pooled clinical sensitivity of RDTs was 72.3% (95% CI: 67.9–76.4), but specificity was 99.8% (95% CI: 99.5–99.9), compared to a pooled clinical sensitivity and specificity of 92.6% (95% CI: 89.8, 94.8) and 99.6% (95% CI: 99, 99.9), respectively, among HIV-negative persons. Possible explanations for this reduced sensitivity include an increased incidence of occult hepatitis B in HIV-positive persons (i.e. presence of HBV DNA with undetectable HBsAg levels, such that HBsAg might not be detected using the RDTs evaluated), and the use of tenofovir- or lamivudine-based antiretroviral regimens, which are active against HBV and may suppress HBV DNA and HBsAg levels. In the one study *(214)* that evaluated three EIAs against an EIA reference with neutralization, the overall pooled sensitivity in HIV-positive individuals was 97.9% (95% CI: 96.0–99.0) and specificity was 99.4% (95% CI: 99.0–99.7), suggesting that EIAs perform better in HIV-positive persons.

Analytical sensitivity/limit of detection. The analytical sensitivity or limit of detection (LoD) is another important performance criteria, but there were insufficient data in the included studies to undertake a systematic comparison. However, no RDTs met the levels of analytical sensitivity (i.e. LoD of 0.130 IU/mL) required by the European Union through its Common Technical Specifications. Data from WHO prequalification assessment studies indicate that the LoD of EIAs for HBsAg was 50–100-fold better compared to RDTs *(230)*. However, despite this difference in analytical sensitivity, clinical sensitivity is unlikely to be greatly reduced because the vast majority of chronic HBV infection is associated with blood HBsAg concentrations well over 10 IU/mL. This is important, as it has been suggested that false-negative RDTs for HBsAg are due to low HBsAg viral load levels, the presence of HBsAg mutants or specific genotypes, and the use of lamivudine- or tenofovir-based ART regimens *(208, 214, 216, 230)*.

The overall quality of the evidence for the recommendation of which serological assay to use was rated as low to moderate, with downgrading mainly due to serious risk of bias based on cross-sectional study design, and heterogeneity in results.

TABLE 7.1. Summary test accuracy of RDTs and EIAs for HBsAg (different assay formats and comparators, populations and specimen types)

Comparison	Pooled sensitivity (95% CI)	Pooled specificity (95% CI)
Assay format and comparators		
RDT versus EIA (*N*=30)	90.0 (89.1–90.8)	99.5 (99.4–99.5)
EIA versus another EIA (*N*=5)	88.9 (87–90.6)	98.4 (97.8–98.8)
RDT versus NAT (*N*=3)	93.3 (91.3–94.9)	98.1 (97–98.9)
RDT versus CMIA (*N*=5)	80.4 (77.9–82.6)	99.0 (99.6–99.3)
Population (RDT versus EIA)		
Blood donors (*N*=7)	91.6 (90.1–92.9)	99.5 (99.3–99.7)
HIV positive (*N*=5)	72.3 (67.9–76.4)	99.8 (99.5–99.9)
HIV negative (*N*=1)	92.6 (89.8–94.8)	99.6 (99.0–99.9)
RDT kit brand (RDT versus EIA)		
Determine HBsAg (*N*=10)	90.8 (88.9–92.4)	99.1 (98.9–99.4)
BinaxNOW HBsAg (*N*=3)	97.6 (96.2–98.6)	100 (99.7–100)
VIKIA HBsAg (*N*=3)	82.5 (77.5–86.7)	99.9 (99.8–100)
Serodia HBsAg (*N*=3)	82.5 (77.5–86.7)	99.9 (99.8–100)
Specimen type (RDT)		
Capillary whole blood versus serum (*N*=8)	91.7 (89.1–93.9)	99.9 (99.8–99.9)

CMIA: chemiluminiscent microparticle immunoassay; EIA: enzyme immunoassay; RDT: rapid diagnostic test

Which testing strategy to use

No studies were identified that directly compared the diagnostic accuracy of a one- versus two-assay serological testing strategy in high- and low-prevalence settings (see *Web annex 5.5*). A predictive modelling analysis was therefore undertaken, which examined diagnostic accuracy of a one- or two-assay strategy based on a hypothetical population of 1000 individuals across both a range of HBsAg seroprevalence levels (10%, 2%, 0.4% representing typical high-, medium- and low-seroprevalence settings or populations, respectively) and a range of assay performance characteristics (sensitivity of 98% and 90%, and specificity of 99% and 98% derived from the systematic review pooled sensitivity and specificity for HBsAg RDTs.

Prevalence had a strong impact on the PPV and the ratio of true-positive to false-positive results (see *Web annex 6.1*). The introduction of a second assay of similar sensitivity to be applied to all specimens reactive in the initial serological assay provides substantial potential gains in the PPV across all prevalence levels (>97%), but particularly at a low prevalence (0.4%) and with an assay that has a lower specificity.

The overall quality of the evidence for the recommendation on use of a one- or two-assay serological testing strategy was rated as low, as this was based on predictive modelling simulation and hypothetical scenarios.

7.4. Rationale for the recommendations on which assay to use

The Guidelines Development Group recognized the critical need to expand testing to identify as many persons as possible with chronic HBV infection who might benefit the most from antiviral treatment and other interventions, and therefore made strong recommendations for a simplified one-assay testing strategy using either EIA or RDTs. Overall, the selection of assay format (EIA[3] or RDT) to test for HBsAg in a particular setting will depend first on the performance characteristics of the assay, but also on key operational considerations, such as accessibility, cost, ease of use in the intended-use setting i.e. technical complexity of test procedure and specimen collection methods. The most sensitive assay available, either RDT or EIA, in terms of clinical sensitivity, should be used.

Balance of benefits and harms

Use of EIAs. In settings where existing laboratory testing infrastructure is available and there is good access to laboratory services, EIAs were recommended as the preferred testing method for several reasons:

1. Although RDTs and EIAs for HBsAg had similar clinical sensitivity and specificity when compared to an EIA reference standard, the sensitivity of different RDTs was highly variable, and some RDTs had suboptimal sensitivity.

2. In HIV-infected individuals, clinical sensitivity of RDTs was poor (72.3%) and appears to be better for EIAs.

3. The analytical sensitivity is much higher for EIAs (50- to 100-fold higher). The benefit of more analytically sensitive assays with better limits of detection is that it improves detection in persons with primary infection, and in individuals in whom HBsAg levels are extremely low.

[3] It is assumed that CLIA and ECL would have similar performance principles as EIAs.

4. A confirmatory test using a neutralization step can be incorporated into laboratory-based EIAs.

5. Testing using laboratory-based EIAs can be automated and may be more appropriate and cost–effective in settings where there are many tests being performed per day (>40 per day per operator).

Use of RDTs

1. The Guidelines Development Group recognized that despite the significant heterogeneity and suboptimal clinical and analytical sensitivity of certain RDTs for HBsAg, expanded use of quality-assured RDTs has a major potential to help scale up HBsAg testing in settings with poor access to or lack of existing laboratory infrastructure to conduct EIAs, such as in remote settings or with hard-to-reach populations.

2. The use of RDTs may be also appropriate in high-income countries to increase the uptake of hepatitis testing in populations that may be reluctant to test or have poor access to health-care services (e.g. PWID) and in outreach programmes (e.g. prison services, harm reduction and drug treatment services).

3. Key challenges to the use of RDTs include the limited availability of quality-assured RDTs for HBsAg detection, reduced analytical sensitivity compared to laboratory-based methods, and that very few HBsAg RDTs meet the analytical sensitivity (LoD 0.130 IU/mL) required by the European Union. However, overall, the Guidelines Development Group considered that the benefits of RDTs in terms of increased access would mitigate potential harms related to lower accuracy, especially if there was careful selection of RDTs that met minimum performance criteria.

In HIV-positive persons, RDTs had low clinical sensitivity (pooled sensitivity of 72.3%). Although this may be potentially explained by the impact of tenofovir- or lamivudine-containing ART regimens, there is a need for caution in their use and interpretation in HIV-positive patients.

Minimum performance criteria for EIAs and RDTs. RDTs for HBsAg have reduced analytical sensitivity and LoD compared to EIAs, as well as wide variation in clinical sensitivity and specificity between assays, and between different studies of the same assay. However, clinical sensitivity is unlikely to be greatly reduced because the vast majority of chronic HBV infection is associated with blood HBsAg concentrations well over 10 IU/mL. However, careful consideration should be given to ensure that the assay chosen has minimal rates of false positivity (both analytical and clinical). The Guidelines Development Group decided against defining minimum performance characteristics for assays, but recommended that any assay used should meet the performance criteria of stringent (see chapter 15) regulatory authorities in terms of both analytical and clinical sensitivity and specificity.

> The recommendations for use of either RDTs or EIAs/CLIAs/ECLs were based on the assumption that all HBsAg assays used should meet minimum performance criteria of either WHO prequalification of IVDs or a stringent regulatory review for IVDs. All IVDs should be used in accordance with manufacturers' instructions for use.

7.5. Rationale for the recommendations on testing strategy

Balance of benefits and harms

When to use a one-assay strategy. A one-assay testing strategy is applicable to most testing settings in resource-limited countries based on simplicity and in populations where prevalence is ≥0.4%, and so PPVs are high.

The Guidelines Development Group made an overall conditional recommendation for a one-assay serological testing strategy to diagnose chronic HBV infection based on low-quality evidence for the following reasons:

1. This approach will efficiently identify (rule in) most individuals likely to be infected and in need of further evaluation, and will rule out those who are uninfected.

2. Although a one-assay serological testing strategy has a lower PPV than a two-assay serological testing strategy, particularly at lower levels of prevalence (0.4% and 2%), and will therefore generate more false-positive results, the Guidelines Development Group considered that the consequences of this would not be clinically significant. This is because all HBsAg-positive patients will have further evaluation with staging of liver disease and HBV DNA measurement to assess eligibility for treatment (i.e. presence of cirrhosis or evidence of raised HBV DNA levels). Therefore, no patient would be initiated on lifelong antiviral therapy on the basis of a single serological test.

3. The Guidelines Development Group noted that it is also common practice in many settings to perform a second test after 6 months to confirm a diagnosis of CHB and so distinguish it from acute hepatitis B. This provides an additional approach to confirm a diagnosis of chronic hepatitis infection.

4. If one uses a first test with high specificity then very few would require a second test.

5. It would considerably simplify the process of testing and reduce costs, especially if delivered at the point of care.

6. More rapid reporting of test results (ideally same day) will help improve access and linkage to care.

When to use a two-assay strategy. The Guidelines Development Group made a conditional recommendation to consider a second serological assay in very low-prevalence settings (<0.4%) to improve the PPV. In low prevalence settings, there will be more false-positive than true-positive results with a single serological assay, even with a test of 99% specificity. Employing two assays with a specificity of around 99% increases the ratio of true-positive to false-positive diagnoses from 0.2 to 32–40.

The recommendation is to confirm with a neutralization step if using laboratory-based immunoassays for detection of HBsAg, as per the assay manufacturer's instructions. Where an RDT for HBsAg is used and no neutralization reagents are available or for EIAs with no neutralization reagents, a second different RDT assay may be used *(231)*. However, there has been limited evaluation of the added value of a second RDT, and there are several challenges: (i) "different" RDT assays may fundamentally be the same, and therefore prone to similar inaccuracies and false-positive reactions; (ii) if the analytical or clinical sensitivity of the assay used is poor (high LoD), then a larger proportion of individuals who are truly HBsAg positive will not be identified, regardless of whether a one- or two-test strategy is used.

Acceptability, values and preferences

In a values and preferences survey among 104 respondents from 43 (20 high-income, 23 low- and middle-income) countries, overall, there was strong support from patient groups for simplified testing strategies that would improve access to testing including for high-risk groups. Seventy-seven per cent expressed a strong preference for a one-serological assay testing strategy with same-day results using RDTs to reduce loss to follow up.

Feasibility

In a survey of programmatic experience with hepatitis testing across 19 LMICs, implementing partners reported widespread use of RDTs in all settings, and use of a single HBsAg RDT assay by 68% of respondents.

Resource considerations

The reagent costs for HBsAg assays are similar for RDTs (between US$ 0.95 and US$ 3.00) and EIAs (between US$ 0.40 and US$ 2.80). High-throughput EIAs require additional laboratory infrastructure and equipment, and precision and expertise in operation. In contrast, RDTs do not require capital investment in laboratory infrastructure, and so there is a concurrent reduction in maintenance costs for equipment.

8. HOW TO TEST FOR CURRENT OR PAST HCV INFECTION (HCV EXPOSURE) – choice of serological assay and testing strategy

8.1. Recommendations

HOW TO TEST FOR CHRONIC HCV INFECTION AND MONITOR TREATMENT RESPONSE	
Topic	**Recommendations**
Which serological assays to use	• To test for serological evidence of past or present infection in adults, adolescents and children (>18 months of age[1]), an HCV serological assay (antibody or antibody/antigen) using either RDT or laboratory-based immunoassay formats[2] that meet minimum safety, quality and performance standards[3] (*with regard to both analytical and clinical sensitivity and specificity*) is recommended. - In settings where there is limited access to laboratory infrastructure and testing, and/or in populations where access to rapid testing would facilitate linkage to care and treatment, RDTs are recommended. *Strong recommendation, low/moderate quality of evidence*
Serological testing strategies	In adults and children older than 18 months[1], a single serological assay for initial detection of serological evidence of past or present infection is recommended prior to supplementary nucleic acid testing (NAT) for evidence of viraemic infection. *Conditional recommendation, low quality of evidence*

Abbreviations: DBS: dried blood spot; IVD: in vitro diagnostics; NAT: nucleic acid test; RDT: rapid diagnostic test

[1] HCV infection can be confirmed in children under 18 months only by virological assays to detect HCV RNA, because transplacental maternal antibodies remain in the child's bloodstream up until 18 months of age, making test results from serology assays ambiguous.

[2] Laboratory-based immunoassays include enzyme immunoassay (EIA), chemoluminescence immunoassay (CLIA), and electrochemoluminescence assay (ECL).

[3] Assays should meet minimum acceptance criteria of either WHO prequalification of IVDs or a stringent regulatory review for IVDs. All IVDs should be used in accordance with manufacturers' instructions, and where possible at testing sites enrolled in a national or international external quality assessment scheme. A lower level of analytical sensitivity can be considered, if an assay is able to improve access (i.e. an assay that can be used at the point of care or suitable for dried blood spot [DBS] specimens) and/or affordability. An assay with a limit of detection of 3000 IU/mL or lower would be acceptable and would identify 95% of those with viraemic infection, based on available data.

FIG. 8.1. WHO-recommended single-assay testing strategy for detection of HCV antibody, irrespective of prevalence

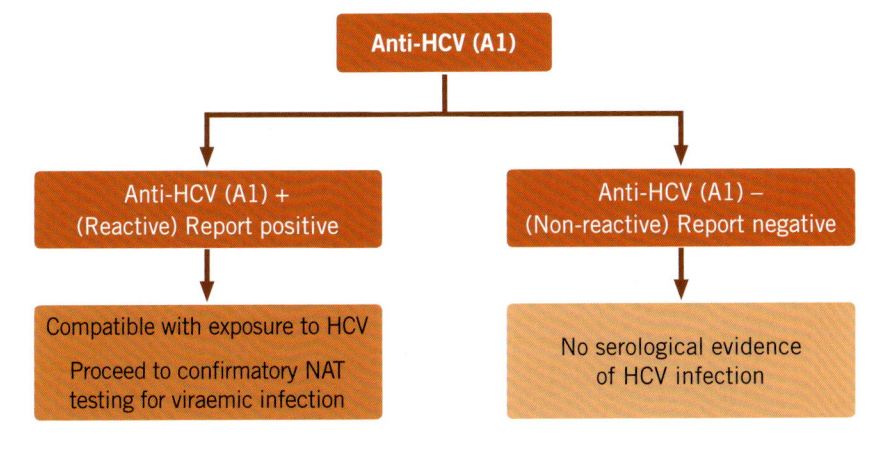

```
                    Anti-HCV (A1)
                   /              \
    Anti-HCV (A1) +              Anti-HCV (A1) –
   (Reactive) Report positive    (Non-reactive) Report negative
           |                              |
   Compatible with exposure to HCV     No serological evidence
   Proceed to confirmatory NAT          of HCV infection
   testing for viraemic infection
```

8.2. Background

The principal assays used to determine exposure to HCV infection and evidence of past or current HCV infection rely on detection of antibodies to HCV using relatively inexpensive serological assays. Such antibody-based assays are unable to detect infection soon after acquisition of HCV infection, as antibodies may not be detected for 2–3 months in an individual who has been recently infected *(135)*. This diagnostic window period can be shortened by using assays that also directly detect HCV antigen. Assessing HCV exposure typically involves either a one- or two-serological assay testing strategy. The main rationale for the use of a second HCV antibody test is to minimize false-positive results and reduce the number of people referred for more costly NAT technologies to confirm viraemic HCV infection. If HCV antibody positivity is established consistent with past or current infection, testing for current viraemic HCV infection is performed to ascertain viral replication through the detection of HCV RNA or HCV (p22) core antigen (HCVcAg). Aside from blood and organ donation screening, HCV RNA is not currently used to determine exposure to HCV, in spite of the shorter window period (1–2 weeks after the onset of acute infection) primarily for reasons of access and cost *(135)*.

8.3. Summary of the evidence

Which serological assay to use

A systematic review (see *Web annex 5.4*) compared the diagnostic performance (sensitivity, specificity, positive and negative predictive values) of commercially available serological assays (RDTs and EIAs) for the detection of HCV antibody, when compared to a laboratory-based immunoassay reference standard. Five studies evaluated RDTs compared to an EIA reference *(201, 232–235)*, 13 studies compared RDT results to NAT or immunoblot *(236–248)* and 14 studies compared RDTs with a combination of EIA, immunoblot or NAT *(197, 201, 232–235, 247, 249–255)*. Twelve studies compared RDTs using oral fluid to RDTs using whole blood (as well as serum or plasma) *(235, 238, 240, 241, 246–248, 250, 251, 255–257)*. The studies were carried out on different source populations, including the general population, key populations and hospital patients. The sample sizes of the included studies ranged from 37 to 17 894. All studies used a cross-sectional or case–control design.

RDTs. Based on the five studies of RDTs compared to EIA-only reference standard, the pooled RDT sensitivity and specificity were, respectively, 99% (95% CI: 98–100) and 100% (95% CI: 100–100), but sensitivities in individual studies ranged from 83% to 100%, and specificities from 99% to 100%.

Brands. There was significant heterogeneity between studies and variable performance across RDT brands and even within the same brand. Although use of NAT or immunoblot is not an appropriate reference to assess RDT diagnostic performance, the pooled sensitivity and specificity of RDTs were 93% (95% CI: 91–95%) and 98% (95% CI: 97–99%), respectively (Table 8.1).

Populations. A high sensitivity (>95%) and specificity (>99%) of RDTs for HCV antibody were observed across populations screened (general population, key populations, hospital patients) using different reference standards (EIA, immunoblot), but a patient selection bias was evident in around a third of studies.

Specimen type. RDTs using oral fluid showed a lower sensitivity but higher specificity compared to the reference standard, respectively, at 94% (95% CI: 93–96%) and 100% (95% CI: 100–100%). However, eight studies that examined OraQuick ADVANCE® HCV Rapid Antibody Test (OraSure Technologies, Inc.) had a higher sensitivity of 98% (95% CI: 97–98) compared to the other brands examined in six studies (pooled sensitivity of 88% [95% CI: 84–92]). There were insufficient data for other key brands, including the SD-Bioline which is now WHO prequalified.

RDTs and EIAs in HIV-positive persons. The number of studies was insufficient to undertake subanalyses based on HIV coinfection *(256, 260–263)*. However, one recent study has reported that HCV EIAs may be associated with high rates of false positivity among HIV-infected persons in Africa *(258)*.

The overall quality of the evidence for the recommendation to use RDTs was rated from low to moderate with downgrading mainly due to a serious risk of bias based on cross-sectional study design, and heterogeneity of results.

TABLE 8.1. Summary diagnostic accuracy of HCV antibody tests (different assay format and comparators, populations, specimen type and oral kit brand)

Comparison	Pooled sensitivity (95% CI)	Pooled specificity (95% CI)
Assay format and comparators		
RDT versus EIA only (*N*=5)	99 (98–100)	100 (100–100)
RDT versus NAT or or immunoblot (*N*=13)	93 (91–95)	98 (97–99)
RDT versus EIA, NAT or immunoblot (*N*=14)	97 (96–98)	100 (100–100)
Antibody and antigen combo testing (*N*=6)	86 (79–94)	99 (98–100)
Populations (RDT versus EIA, NAT or immunoblot)		
General population (*N*=17)	95 (94–96)	99 (98–99)
Key populations (*N*=19)	97 (96–98)	94 (94–95)
Hospital patients (*N*=16)	97 (96–98)	100 (100–100)
Specimen type (RDT vs EIA, NAT or immunoblot)		
Blood specimens (*N*=45)	98 (97–98)	98 (98–99)
Oral fluid specimens (*N*=12)	94 (93–96)	100 (100–100)
Oral RDT versus blood reference (*N*=12)	94 (93–96)	99.9 (99.8–100)
Oral kit brands		
OraQuick (*N*=8)	98 (97–99)	100 (100–100)
Other brands (Chembio DPP, Blioeasy, ImmunoComb II (*N*=6)	88 (84–92)	99 (99–100)

EIA: enzyme immunoassay; NAT: nucleic acid test; RDT: rapid diagnostic test

Which testing strategy to use

There was a single cost-effectiveness analysis that compared three testing strategies in a Brazilian population *(259) (*see *Web annex 5.6)*. They found that a one-serological assay testing strategy for detection of anti-HCV followed by HCV RNA NAT to establish viraemic HCV infection was more cost–effective than a two-serological assay testing strategy. A predictive modelling study was also undertaken, which examined the diagnostic accuracy of a one- or two-assay HCV antibody testing strategy based on a hypothetical population of 1000 individuals across both a range of HCV antibody seroprevalence levels that reflect typical high prevalence rates among PWID [45%], intermediate prevalence among HIV-infected MSM [10%] and moderate [2%] to low [0.4%] endemicity in a general population), and across a range of assay performance characteristics (sensitivity of 98% and 90%, and specificity of 99% and 98% derived from the systematic review pooled sensitivity and specificity for HCV antibody RDTs, Table 8.1).

The outcomes show the strong influence of prevalence and assay specificity on PPV (*see Web annex 6.2*). The use of a highly sensitive and specific (98% and 99%) single assay yields a high PPV in excess of 90% at prevalences of 40% and 10%, and 67% at a 2% prevalence, and only a small number of false-positive diagnoses. Only at the lowest prevalence (e.g. 0.4%) does the PPV fall below 50%. Since overall the PPV is high at all prevalence levels with a single assay, the use of a second test would have a significant impact only in the lowest-prevalence populations (0.4%), especially if the initial assay was of lower performance.

8.4. Rationale for the recommendations on which assay to use

Overall, the Guidelines Development Group made a strong recommendation for the use of serological assays, particularly RDTs, based on moderate/low-quality evidence for diagnostic performance. As for HBsAg, the selection of assay format (either EIA[4] or RDT) to test for HCV antibody in a particular setting will depend first on the performance characteristics of the assay, cost and also on key operational considerations, such as accessibility and ease of use in the intended-use setting, such as a community-based drug treatment programme versus a hospital-based clinic.

Balance of benefits and harms

Use of RDTs. In settings where access to laboratory services is limited, or where existing testing services do not have the capacity for conducting EIA, and for hard-to-reach and rural populations, the Guidelines Development Group recommended (as for HIV and HBsAg) the use of quality-assured RDTs rather than conventional laboratory-based EIAs. This was due mainly to their simplicity, relatively low cost and rapid turnaround time, and therefore their potential to substantially improve access to HCV testing, enhance linkage to care and reduce loss to follow up.

Other reasons for the preferred use of RDTs include the following:

1. RDTs for the detection of antibodies to HCV have acceptable sensitivity and specificity compared to laboratory-based EIAs across a wide range of settings and different populations and for different brands. RDTs that use oral fluid are also available, which have adequate sensitivity and specificity, and may therefore be particularly useful where collection of venous or capillary whole blood is challenging.

2. RDTs performed at the point of care, using less invasively collected specimens than venous whole blood, may allow for results to be available on the same day as testing, and so avoid the need for multiple follow-up appointments and reduce loss to follow up.

3. For national programmes in resource-limited settings, expanded use of RDTs may mitigate the challenges of specimen collection, processing and transportation to laboratory services, and allow for the simplification and decentralization of testing.

[4] It is assumed that CLIA and ECL would have similar performance principles to EIAs.

4. RDTs can also be used in outreach programmes (e.g. prison services, substance use/treatment services) in HICs to increase the uptake of hepatitis screening. Well-trained community health workers can perform testing accurately and reliably.

Use of EIAs. In settings with existing laboratory infrastructure or where many tests are carried out per day, testing by laboratory-based methods, such as EIAs, may be cost–effective and appropriate.

Although RDTs and EIAs had similar clinical sensitivity and specificity, testing using laboratory-based EIAs was recommended as the more appropriate and cost–effective assay in settings where suitable laboratory infrastructure is available, and where there is likely to be high-volume throughput, with many tests performed per day (>40 per day per operator), and in individuals who have good access to laboratory-based testing.

It is important to note that the latest generation of assays designed to detect HCV antibody are also designed to detect HCVcAg in order to increase the sensitivity of the assay and reduce the diagnostic window period. However, these fourth-generation assays are not typically able to differentiate HCV exposure from chronic HCV infection.

In HIV-positive persons. Insufficient studies were retrieved for the systematic review of persons with HIV/HCV coinfection for a formal evaluation of the diagnostic accuracy of RDTs to detect antibodies to HCV in persons who are HIV coinfected. Theoretically, the sensitivity of serological assays that detect antibodies only may be reduced if the patient is immunocompromised, e.g. persons with HIV infection, those undergoing immunosuppressive therapy or renal dialysis, and therefore exposure to HCV may not be detected in these individuals. It is estimated that this may occur in up to 6% of HIV-infected persons who undergo testing using an EIA for the detection of antibodies to HCV *(260, 261)* but may occur more often among persons with advanced immunosuppression due to HIV and during early HCV infection *(262, 263)*. Conversely, there are also reports of a large proportion of false-positive HCV serological tests among HIV-infected persons, especially in SSA *(258)*.

Minimum performance criteria for EIAs and RDTs. The Guidelines Development Group decided against defining minimum performance characteristics for assays, but recommended that any assay used should meet the performance criteria for stringent regulatory authorities (*see* Chapter 15). The Group also recognized that performance of RDTs in the field (i.e. setting of intended use) may vary and that certain RDTs are not validated by the manufacturer for use on capillary whole blood. The issues of analytical sensitivity and LoD for HCV antibody assays is less relevant than for HBsAg for several reasons. First, there are no WHO reference standard materials for anti-HCV antibody, and so IU/mL cannot be applied. Second, in contrast to the 40–100-fold difference in LoD for HBsAg detection, there is a minimal difference in end-point titres for anti-HCV antibody between RDTs and EIAs.

> The recommendations for the use of either RDTs or EIAs/CLIAs/ECLs were based on the assumption that all HCV antibody assays used should meet minimum performance criteria of either WHO prequalification of IVDs or a stringent regulatory review for IVDs. All IVDs should be used in accordance with manufacturers' instructions for use.

8.5. Rationale for the recommendation for a one-assay serological testing strategy

Balance of benefits and harms

The Guidelines Development Group made a conditional recommendation for a single test using an RDT or EIA, followed by HCV RNA NAT or core antigen on reactive specimens as the simplest and most feasible testing strategy in all settings based on low-quality evidence for several reasons.

1. Predictive modelling indicates that a one-assay testing strategy efficiently identifies all but a very few individuals likely to be infected and in need of NAT testing to confirm viraemic HCV infection, and similarly excludes nearly all HCV-uninfected individuals, even at low prevalence. The overall impact of the second assay on improving PPV was smaller compared to the situation with HBsAg because of the generally higher sensitivity and specificity of RDTs for HCV antibody.

2. There are concerns about the cost implications and feasibility of implementing a second serological assay, particularly at the point of care and in resource-limited settings.

3. In low-prevalence populations, a higher proportion of results would be false positive, and therefore individuals would undergo unnecessary and more expensive NAT to identify viraemic infection as a result of a single falsely reactive serological assay. In this situation, the two-assay serological testing strategy may be marginally cost saving. However, the Guidelines Development Group did not consider that the numbers of false-positive diagnoses were significant enough to justify a two-assay serological testing strategy. It was also recognized that many countries in SSA will fall into the low-seroprevalence category of less than 0.4%, and higher rates of false positivity have also been reported in these settings. As access to NAT remains very limited and costly at present, the use of a second serological test may be more cost–effective than performing NATs in multiple persons with false-positive results.

4. The risks associated with a false positive HCV antibody result is minimal, as all individuals with a diagnosis of HCV exposure (HCV seropositive) will require supplemental testing to confirm viraemic HCV infection (by NAT to detect HCV RNA or serology to detect HCVcAg) before initiation of antiviral treatment.

Acceptability, values and preferences

The values and preferences survey showed strong support by the majority for the use of RDTs delivered at the point of care to promote access, and a simplified one-serological assay testing strategy for HCV exposure, followed by supplementary testing to detect viraemic HCV infection. Providers and patients found RDTs that utilize oral fluid specimens to be more acceptable than capillary or venous whole blood specimens, especially in children.[5]

Resource use

The cost of RDTs for HCV antibodies ranges from US$ 0.50 to US$ 2.00 for blood-based assays, and US$ 10 for oral fluid RDTs. The cost of EIAs ranges from US$ 0.50 to US$ 1.70, but EIAs require additional laboratory infrastructure and equipment, with precision and expertise required in their operation. RDTs do not require capital investment in laboratory infrastructure, and so there is a concurrent reduction in maintenance costs and reagents. Using a second different RDT assay would at least double the costs.

Feasibility

A survey of hepatitis testing programmatic experience across 19 LMICs found that a one-serological assay testing strategy using mainly RDTs was being implemented in a range of hospital-based services, including blood donor screening, harm-reduction services, and HIV treatment and care clinics.

8.6. Implementation considerations for HBsAg and HCV antibody serological testing

The most sensitive assay available, either RDT or EIA, in terms of both analytical sensitivity and clinical sensitivity, should be used. RDTs generally have a lower analytical sensitivity (IU/mL LoD) compared to EIAs. However, careful consideration should be given to ensure that the assay chosen has minimal rates of false positivity (both analytical and clinical). *See also* Chapter 15 for details on how to set up laboratory services for hepatitis testing and selection of an assay, and how to assure the quality of hepatitis B and hepatitis C testing.

1. **Quality-assured and fit-for-purpose assays.** Access to a range of well-performing quality-assured assays is critical to the success of any hepatitis testing programme. While a wide variety of EIAs (and CLIAs, ECLs) are commercially available, there is a lack of HBsAg RDTs that meet minimum performance criteria, as well as safety and quality standards. National regulatory authorities are responsible for approving RDTs for sale and use after assessment of their quality, safety and performance.

---

[5] Most RDTs using oral fluid are yet to be validated and then evaluated in children.

2. **Accurate testing.** All hepatitis B and C testing should be performed in accordance with the assay manufacturer's instructions, including an HBsAg neutralization step if it is being utilized. In addition, SOPs and job aids can help testing providers minimize testing and reporting errors, and thus improve the quality of the results.

3. **Staff training and supervision.** The testing environment should operate according to quality management systems (*see* Chapter 15), and have access to qualified, proficient and motivated laboratory staff, trained specifically in performance of the various assays, with adequate and supervisory support. Health-care workers should understand the strengths and limitations of any given testing strategy, counsel patients who are screened, and be able to act appropriately on the results, both positive and negative. Delivery of RDTs requires appropriate training of test providers in performing the test, reading the test result, storage of test kits and other supplies, and interpreting and reporting the results.

4. **Linkage to care.** As some preliminary results will be false positive, appropriate linkage will be needed to additional testing and clinical evaluation, especially where testing is conducted at the point of care in outreach programmes. Retesting strategies need to be implemented for those with a high risk of acquisition of HCV.

5. **Provision of NAT or HCVcAg testing** at the same site as serological testing would be optimal, enabling rapid turnaround, reduced loss to follow up, and reduced personal and health-care costs of referral to a distant centre. The Guidelines Development Group did not consider in these guidelines the potential future testing scenario of a single NAT or HCVcAg for both diagnosis and confirmation of active infection.

Research gaps for HBsAg and HCV antibody serological testing

- The impact of HIV positivity (and of CD4 count, viral load and ART exposure, by regimen) on the diagnostic performance of RDTs for HBsAg and HCV antibody should be further evaluated.
- Evaluation should be done of the diagnostic performance, impact, cost and cost–effectiveness of a one- versus two-assay serological HBsAg or HCV testing strategy in diverse settings of both high and low HBsAg and HCV antibody prevalence.
- EIAs and RDTs assays should be validated using less invasive and simpler methods of sample collection, such as oral fluid and capillary whole blood and dried blood spots (DBS).

9. DETECTION OF VIRAEMIC HBV INFECTION – to guide who to treat or not treat

9.1. Recommendation

Detection of HBV DNA – assessment for treatment *Adapted from existing guidance (WHO HBV 2015 guidelines[6])*	• Directly following a positive HBsAg serological test, the use of quantitative or qualitative nucleic acid testing (NAT) for detection of HBV DNA is recommended as the preferred strategy and to guide who to treat or not treat. *Strong recommendation, moderate/low quality of evidence*

Algorithm of WHO recommendations on the management of persons with chronic hepatitis B infection[a]

HBsAg positive

CIRRHOSIS
- Clinical criteria[b]
- NITs (APRI score >2 in adults or FibroScan)

ASSESSMENT FOR TREATMENT

Yes:
- ALL AGES[c] >30 years (in particular)
  - ALT[d,e] Persistently abnormal → HBV DNA >20 000 IU/mL → **INITIATE NA THERAPY AND MONITOR**
    - Tenofovir or entecavir
    - Entecavir in children aged 2–11 years
  - ALT[d,e] Intermittently abnormal → HBV DNA 2000–20 000 IU/mL → DEFER TREATMENT AND MONITOR
  - ALT[d,e] Persistently normal → HBV DNA <2000 IU/mL → DEFER TREATMENT AND MONITOR

No:
- AGE ≤30 years
  - ALT[d,e] Persistently normal → HBV DNA <2000 IU/mL → DEFER TREATMENT AND MONITOR

MONITORING
- Every 6 months: **DETECTION OF HCC[f]** (persons with cirrhosis or HCC family history)
- Every 12 months: **DISEASE PROGRESSION AND/OR TREATMENT RESPONSE IN ALL[f]**
- Baseline and every 12 months: **TOXICITY MONITORING IN PERSONS ON TREATMENT** Renal function[g] and risk factors for renal dysfunction

STOPPING TREATMENT
- **CIRRHOSIS** Lifelong treatment
- **NO CIRRHOSIS**
  - and HBeAg loss and seroconversion to anti-HBe and after completion of at least one additional year of treatment
  - and persistently normal ALT
  - and persistently undetectable HBV DNA

NITs: non-invasive tests, ALT: alanine aminotransferase, APRI: aspartate aminotransferase-to-platelet ratio index

[a] Defined as persistence of hepatitis B surface antigen (HBsAg) for six months or more. The algorithm does not capture all potential scenarios, but the main categories for treatment or monitoring. Recommendations for settings without access to HBV DNA testing are provided in the relevant chapters.
[b] Clinical features of decompensated cirrhosis: portal hypertension (ascites, variceal haemorrhage and hepatic encephalopathy), coagulopathy, or liver insufficiency (jaundice). Other clinical features of advanced liver disease/cirrhosis may include: hepatomegaly, splenomegaly, pruritus, fatigue, arthralgia, palmar erythema, and oedema.
[c] The age cut-off of >30 years is not absolute, and some persons with CHB less than 30 years may also meet criteria for antiviral treatment.
[d] ALT levels fluctuate in persons with chronic hepatitis B and require longitudinal monitoring to determine the trend. Upper limits for normal ALT have been defined as below 30 U/L for men and 19 U/L for women, though local laboratory normal ranges should be applied. Persistently normal/abnormal may be defined as three ALT determinations below or above the upper limit of normal, made at unspecified intervals during a 6–12-month period or predefined intervals during 12-month period.
[e] Where HBV DNA testing is not available, treatment may be considered based on persistently abnormal ALT levels, but other common causes of persistently raised ALT levels such as impaired glucose tolerance, dyslipidaemia and fatty liver should be excluded.
[f] All persons with CHB should be monitored regularly for disease activity/progression and detection of HCC, and after stopping treatment for evidence of reactivation. More frequent monitoring maybe required in those with more advanced liver disease, during the first year of treatment or where adherence is a concern, and in those with abnormal ALT and HBV DNA levels >2000 IU/mL, not yet on treatment.
[g] Before initiation, assessment should be done of renal function (serum creatinine level, estimated glomerular filtration rate, urine dipsticks for proteinuria and glycosuria, and risk factors for renal dysfunction [decompensated cirrhosis, CrCl <50 mL/min, poorly controlled hypertension, proteinuria, uncontrolled diabetes, active glomerulonephritis, concomitant nephrotoxic drugs, solid organ transplantation, older age, BMI <18.5 kg/m² (or body weight <50 kg], concomitant use of nephrotoxic drugs or a boosted protease inhibitor [PI] for HIV). Monitoring should be more frequent in those at higher risk of renal dysfunction.

Existing recommendations on Who to treat and not treat (2015 WHO HBV guidelines)

Who to treat

- As a priority, all adults, adolescents and children with CHB[a] and clinical evidence of compensated or decompensated cirrhosis[b] (or cirrhosis based on APRI score >2 in adults) should be treated, regardless of ALT levels, HBeAg status or HBV DNA levels. *(Strong recommendation, moderate quality of evidence)*

- Treatment is recommended for adults with CHB[a] who do not have clinical evidence of cirrhosis (or based on APRI score ≤2 in adults), but are aged more than 30 years[c] (in particular), and have persistently abnormal ALT levels[d,e] and evidence of high-level HBV replication (HBV DNA >20 000 IU/mL[f]), regardless of HBeAg status. *(Strong recommendation, moderate quality of evidence)*

   › Where HBV DNA testing is not available: treatment may be considered based on persistently abnormal ALT levels alone[e], regardless of HBeAg status. *(Conditional recommendation, low quality of evidence)*

Who not to treat but continue to monitor

- Antiviral therapy is not recommended and can be deferred in persons without clinical evidence of cirrhosis (or based on APRI score ≤2 in adults), and with persistently normal ALT levels[d,e] and low levels of HBV replication (HBV DNA <2000 IU/mL[f]), regardless of HBeAg status or age. *(Strong recommendation, low quality of evidence)*

   › Where HBV DNA testing is not available: Treatment can be deferred in HBeAg-positive persons aged 30 years or less and persistently normal ALT levels. *(Conditional recommendation, low quality of evidence)*

- Continued monitoring is necessary in all persons with CHB, but in particular those who do not currently meet the above-recommended criteria for who to treat or not treat, to determine if antiviral therapy may be indicated in the future to prevent progressive liver disease. These include:

- persons without cirrhosis aged 30 years or less, with HBV DNA levels >20 000 IU/ mL[e] but persistently normal ALT;

- HBeAg-negative persons without cirrhosis aged 30 years or less, with HBV DNA levels that fluctuate between 2000 and 20 000 IU/mL, or who have intermittently abnormal ALT levels[d,e];

   › **Where HBV DNA measurement is not available:** persons without cirrhosis aged 30 years or less, with persistently normal or ALT levels, regardless of HBeAg status.

---

[a] Clinical features of decompensated cirrhosis: portal hypertension (ascites, variceal haemorrhage and hepatic encephalopathy), coagulopathy, or liver insufficiency (jaundice). Other clinical features of advanced liver disease/cirrhosis may include: hepatomegaly, splenomegaly, pruritus, fatigue, arthralgia, palmar erythema and oedema.

[b] Defined as persistence of hepatitis B surface antigen (HBsAg) for six months or more

[c] The age cut-off of >30 years is not absolute, and some persons with CHB aged less than 30 years may also meet the criteria for antiviral treatment.

[d] ALT levels fluctuate in persons with CHB and require longitudinal monitoring to determine the trend. Upper limits for normal ALT have been defined as below 30 U/L for men and 19 U/L for women (based on greater sensitivity observed in hepatitis B for histological disease in the liver), though local laboratory normal ranges should be applied. Persistently normal/abnormal may be defined as three ALT determinations below or above the upper limit of normal, made at unspecified intervals during a 6–12-month period or predefined intervals during a 12-month period.

[e] Where HBV DNA testing is not available, other common causes of persistently raised ALT levels such as impaired glucose tolerance, dyslipidaemia and fatty liver should be excluded.

[f] WHO has defined an international standard for expression of HBV DNA concentrations. Serum HBV DNA levels should be expressed in IU/mL to ensure comparability; the same assay should be used in the same patient to evaluate antiviral efficacy. All HBV DNA values in the recommendations are reported in IU/mL; values given as copies/mL were converted to IU/mL after dividing by a factor of 5 (10 000 copies/mL = 2000 IU/mL; 100 000 copies/mL = 20 000 IU/mL; 1 million copies/mL =200 000 IU/mL).

Occasionally, extrahepatic manifestations of hepatitis B, including glomerulonephritis or vasculitis, may be indications for treatment.

9.2 Background

The decision to initiate antiviral therapy is usually based on a combined assessment of the stage of liver disease (from clinical features, and now increasingly from blood or ultrasound-based NITs), together with levels of serum ALT and HBV DNA. Serum HBV DNA concentration quantified by real-time polymerase chain reaction (PCR) measures the extent of viral replication and correlates with disease progression *(264–266)*. It is used to differentiate active HBeAg-negative disease from inactive chronic infection, and inform decisions on treatment and subsequent monitoring.

The objective of treatment is to prevent the adverse outcomes of CHB. The decision to treat is usually clear in persons who present with life-threatening or advanced liver disease, such as acute liver failure, compensated or decompensated cirrhosis, and acute-on-chronic liver failure. However, in persons who have not yet progressed to cirrhosis, it is important that antiviral therapy is targeted to the stage of CHB when the risk of disease progression (fibrosis) is greatest while those persons with minimal fibrosis and low risk of CHB progression that do not require antiviral therapy are identified. Decisions are generally based on ALT and HBV DNA levels. However, not all persons will have raised ALT and HBV DNA levels. For example, during the immune-tolerant phase of disease, there will be high levels of HBV DNA but low or normal levels of ALT, and little liver inflammation or progression of fibrosis. Later on, during the immune-active phase, HBV DNA levels will be low, but ALT levels will be raised, with a much higher risk of disease progression to fibrosis.

9.3. Rationale for the recommendations on HBV DNA measurement (WHO 2015 HBV guidelines)

The Guidelines Development Group recognized that access to HBV DNA measurement remains limited in LMICs. In the 2015 HBV guidelines *(6)*, a strong recommendation was made for use of HBV DNA NAT (quantitative or qualitative) as the most important assay to guide decisions about who to treat or not treat. This was based on low/moderate-quality evidence from 22 observational studies (including four large population-based prospective cohort studies) to identify individuals with the highest and lowest risk of progression (i.e. cirrhosis and HCC) *(Web appendix 2: SRs 5a and 5b – WHO HBV guidelines 2015, http://apps.who.int/iris/bitstream/10665/154590/1/9789241549059_eng.pdf?ua=1&ua=1)*. There are caveats to the generalizability of the evidence. The majority of the studies were from Asia, and there were no data from cohorts in SSA or Latin America, and the data from the REVEAL study may not apply to those with adult-acquired HBV infection, those aged <30 or >65 years, and those infected with HBV genotypes non-B or C. There were also no studies in pregnant women, children or adolescents with CHB.

Balance of benefits and harms

Who to treat

In the 2015 HBV guidelines, it was recommended that antiviral therapy be prioritized for those with life-threatening liver disease (decompensated cirrhosis) and compensated cirrhosis, identified either clinically or using NITs (APRI score based on the single high cut-off >2 for cirrhosis in adults, or FibroScan®), regardless of ALT or HBV DNA levels. In persons who had not progressed to cirrhosis (APRI score ≤2 in adults), it was recommended to target treatment to those at highest risk of disease progression based on the detection of persistently abnormal ALT and HBV DNA levels >20 000 IU/mL (especially in those aged >30 years, regardless of HBeAg status). The recommended thresholds were derived from consistent evidence from large population-based cohort studies of increased risk of HCC and liver cirrhosis above these thresholds. It was recognized that there were uncertainties in the specific thresholds of age, HBV DNA and serum ALT levels for identifying significant fibrosis and/or necroinflammation.

Who not to treat

Conversely, treatment was not recommended in persons with minimal liver disease or fibrosis, and at low risk of progression to cirrhosis and HCC on the basis of persistently normal ALT levels and low levels of HBV replication (<2000 IU/mL), and an APRI score ≤2, as the potential harms of long-term antiviral therapy outweigh the benefits. Long-term monitoring of these persons is required.

In settings where HBV DNA testing is not available

The current limited access to HBV DNA testing in many LMICs is a significant impediment to the effective management of CHB in these settings, and this means that decisions to start treatment will be based on clinical features and serum ALT levels alone.

Overall, there was a very limited evidence base to guide recommendations in the absence of HBV DNA levels, and two conditional recommendations were made in the 2015 WHO HBV guidelines based mainly on expert opinion. First, treatment should be initiated in persons with persistently abnormal ALT levels (regardless of HBeAg status), but where other common causes of persistently abnormal ALT such as impaired glucose tolerance, dyslipidaemia and fatty liver have been excluded. Conversely, treatment was not recommended in HBeAg-negative persons without cirrhosis aged less than 30 years with persistently normal ALT levels. It was recognized that there are several other categories of persons with CHB who do not meet the criteria for initiating or not initiating treatment, who would also require continued monitoring and observation.

9.4. Implementation considerations

- Access to HBV DNA testing is currently very limited in most LMICs, and is a significant impediment to the effective management of CHB in these settings.
- Serum HBV DNA levels should be expressed in IU/mL to ensure comparability; values given as copies/mL can be converted to IU/mL by dividing by a factor of 5 to approximate the conversion used in the most commonly used assays (i.e. 10 000 copies/mL = 2000 IU/mL; 100 000 copies/mL = 20 000 IU/mL; 1 million copies/mL = 200 000 IU/mL).

10. MONITORING FOR HBV TREATMENT RESPONSE AND DISEASE PROGRESSION

10.1. Recommendations

Monitoring for HBV treatment response and disease progression *Existing guidance (WHO HBV 2015 guidelines[1])*	• **It is recommended that the following be monitored at least annually:** – ALT levels (and AST for APRI), HBsAg[2], HBeAg[3], and HBV DNA levels (where HBV DNA testing is available) – Non-invasive tests (APRI score or transient elastography) to assess for presence of cirrhosis in those without cirrhosis at baseline; – If on treatment, adherence should be monitored regularly and at each visit. *Strong recommendation, moderate quality of evidence* **More frequent monitoring is recommended:** • **In persons on treatment or following treatment discontinuation:** more frequent on-treatment monitoring (at least every 3 months for the first year) is indicated in: persons with more advanced disease (compensated or decompensated cirrhosis[4]); during the first year of treatment to assess treatment response and adherence; where treatment adherence is a concern; in HIV-coinfected persons; and in persons after discontinuation of treatment. *Conditional recommendation, very low quality of evidence* • **In persons who do not yet meet the criteria for antiviral therapy:** i.e. persons who have intermittently abnormal ALT levels or HBV DNA levels that fluctuate between 2000 IU/mL and 20 000 IU/mL (where HBV DNA testing is available) and in HIV-coinfected persons[7]. *Conditional recommendation, low quality of evidence*

Abbreviations: ALT: alanine aminotransferase; AST: aspartate aminotransferase; APRI: aspartate-to-platelet ratio index; HBeAg: HBV e antigen; HBsAg: HBV surface antigen; NAT: nucleic acid test; RDT: rapid diagnostic test

[1] For further details, *see* Chapter 5: Who to treat and who not to treat. Guidelines for the prevention, care and treatment of persons with chronic hepatitis B infection: World Health Organization; 2015.
[2] In persons on treatment, monitor for HBsAg loss (although this occurs rarely), and for seroreversion to HBsAg positivity after discontinuation of treatment.
[3] Monitoring of HBeAg/anti-HBe mainly applies to those who are initially HBeAg positive. However, those who have already achieved HBeAg seroconversion and are HBeAg negative and anti-HBe positive may serorevert.
[4] Decompensated cirrhosis is defined by the development of portal hypertension (ascites, variceal haemorrhage and hepatic encephalopathy), coagulopathy, or liver insufficiency (jaundice). Other clinical features of advanced liver disease/cirrhosis may include: hepatomegaly, splenomegaly, pruritus, fatigue, arthralgia, palmar erythema and oedema.

10.2. Background

Prior to treatment

The goal of monitoring HBV DNA and other markers is to identify progression of disease and when to initiate therapy. This can be ascertained by longitudinal monitoring of ALT, HBeAg and HBV DNA levels, where available. Fluctuations or persistently abnormal serum ALT and HBV DNA levels >20 000 IU/mL can indicate progressive disease and the need for treatment. Conversely, spontaneous improvement may occur with a decline in HBV replication, with normalization of ALT levels and seroconversion from HBeAg-positive to anti-HBe. This confers a good prognosis and does not require treatment. Similarly, persons with inactive disease, who are HBeAg-negative with normal ALT levels and low HBV DNA levels (previously called inactive HBsAg carriers), require regular monitoring of HBV DNA and ALT levels to ensure that they remain inactive carriers or, to determine the timing for treatment initiation, any increase in ALT or HBV DNA levels, or evidence of progression to cirrhosis.

During and after treatment

Monitoring while on treatment is required to assess adherence, evaluate whether viral suppression is sustained (where HBV DNA can be measured), assess the potential for treatment discontinuation, and progression of liver disease, including development of HCC. Monitoring after treatment is important to check for reactivation early on and when to restart treatment.

10.3. Rationale for the recommendations (WHO 2015 HBV guidelines)

The optimal timing and frequency of monitoring for serological markers (HBeAg, serum ALT) and HBV DNA to ascertain alterations in disease patterns prior to treatment, as well as assess treatment response have not been well established, and the evidence base is limited. Since no studies had directly compared different monitoring approaches and frequency of monitoring, and there was only indirect evidence from cohort studies, and imprecision due to few events, the quality of evidence was rated as low or very low (*Web appendix 2: SR5a* – WHO HBV guidelines 2015) http://apps.who.int/iris/bitstream/10665/154590/1/9789241549059_eng.pdf?ua=1&ua=1) *(6)*.

Balance of benefits and harms

Monitoring prior to treatment

The 2015 HBV guidelines *(6)* recommended at least annual monitoring of HBV DNA levels, HBeAg and serum ALT to determine any persistent abnormality in ALT or HBV DNA levels (i.e. HBV DNA threshold above >20 000 IU/mL and ALT levels) consistent with risk of disease progression, as well as for development of cirrhosis (based on clinical features or on NITs [APRI >2 in adults]), which would be an indication for antiviral therapy. Additional monitoring of HBeAg may be helpful for several reasons: it indicates the presence of active HBV replication and high infectivity, and spontaneous improvement may occur following HBeAg-positive seroconversion (anti-HBe), with a decline in HBV replication and normalization of ALT levels. This confers a good prognosis and does not require treatment. More frequent monitoring was recommended conditionally (based on limited evidence) in those who already have fluctuating raised ALT or HBV DNA levels (between 2000 IU/mL and 20 000 IU/mL) as they are at a higher risk of progression to active hepatitis and require treatment.

Monitoring during and after treatment

The 2015 WHO HBV guidelines *(6)* recommended at least annual monitoring of ALT, HBeAg (for seroconversion to anti-HBe) and HBV DNA levels (where testing is available), and also NITs such as APRI to assess for progression to cirrhosis. HBV genotyping and resistance testing are not required to guide therapy. This was based on limited data from systematic reviews of multiple clinical trials and observational studies as the minimum and optimal frequency for monitoring treatment response during therapy have not been directly evaluated (*Web appendix 2: SR5a* – WHO HBV guidelines 2015). This shows that potent nucleos(t)ide analogues (NAs) with a high barrier to resistance (i.e. tenofovir and entecavir) suppress HBV DNA replication to low or undetectable levels in the majority of persons (around 80% and 50–70% in HBeAg-positive and -negative persons, respectively) by 24–48 weeks of treatment, with low rates of resistance. The data also suggest that if good adherence can be confirmed, monitoring can be relatively infrequent. However, there is limited success in achieving durable end-points, particularly loss of HBeAg in HBeAg-positive persons or loss of HBsAg.

More frequent and careful monitoring was recommended conditionally based on limited evidence in: (i) those with more advanced disease (compensated or decompensated cirrhosis) because the risk of HCC is reduced but not eliminated with treatment, and their higher risk of adverse events; (ii) during the first year of treatment to assess treatment response; (iii) where adherence to therapy is a concern; and (iv) after stopping therapy, especially in the first year to detect severe exacerbations. Retreatment is recommended if there are consistent signs of reactivation (HBsAg or HBeAg becomes positive, ALT levels increase, or HBV DNA becomes detectable again).

10.4. Implementation considerations

There are cost implications to regular ALT and DNA monitoring. Where there is limited access to HBV DNA assays, such as in LMICs (particularly rural areas), monitoring will require, at a minimum, serum ALT levels to establish the risk of progression. However, interpretation of disease stage and exacerbations of disease in HBeAg-positive and HBeAg-negative persons is enhanced by concomitant measurement of HBV DNA concentrations. Integrating routine monitoring for HCC alongside routine monitoring for disease progression provides a further opportunity to detect the development of cirrhosis and initiate antiviral therapy to prevent progression to HCC or liver failure.

11. DETECTION OF VIRAEMIC HCV INFECTION – to guide who to treat

11.1. Recommendations

Detection of viraemic infection	• Directly following a reactive HCV antibody serological test result, the use of quantitative or qualitative NAT for detection of HCV RNA is recommended as the preferred strategy to diagnose viraemic infection. *Strong recommendation, moderate/low quality of evidence* • An assay to detect HCV core (p22) antigen, which has comparable clinical sensitivity to NAT, is an alternative to NAT to diagnose viraemic infection[1]. *Conditional recommendation, moderate quality of evidence*

[1] A lower level of analytical sensitivity can be considered if an assay is able to improve access (i.e. an assay that can be used at the point of care or suitable for dried blood spot [DBS] specimens) and/or affordability. An assay with a limit of detection of 3000 IU/mL or lower would be acceptable and would identify 95% of those with viraemic infection, based on available data.

11.2. Background

Detection of antibodies to HCV is used to determine current or past HCV infection (i.e. exposure to HCV infection), and therefore to triage those who require further evaluation to determine if active viral replication is present. Approximately 15–45% of persons who are infected with HCV will spontaneously clear the infection *(267)*. These persons remain HCV antibody positive but are no longer infected with HCV. Diagnosis of viraemic HCV infection in those who are HCV antibody positive will distinguish persons with viraemic HCV infection and in need of treatment from those who have cleared the infection. This is generally done using NAT technologies to detect HCV RNA, but an alternative and potentially less costly option to NAT is to conduct testing to detect HCV core (p22) antigen.

Nucleic acid testing (NAT)

Both quantitative and qualitative methods are available for the detection of viraemic HCV infection. Quantitative NAT has been widely used for measuring viral load and identifying those in need of treatment, as well as in assessing treatment response *(5, 15)*. Qualitative NAT allows for rapid and sensitive detection of the virus as well as evidence of a decline in viral RNA level below a defined threshold. There are currently five quantitative HCV RNA (viral load) assays that are commercially available with another two in the pipeline *(268)*. At present, there has been limited comparison of the two methods. Although NAT technologies are very sensitive and specific for the detection of viraemia, they require sophisticated laboratory equipment and skilled staff. Assays to detect HCV RNA that may be used at or near the point of care have recently become commercially available. A comprehensive review of the HCV diagnostics landscapes by UNITAID is available *(268)*.

HCV core (p22) antigen testing

In addition to NAT, it is possible to assess for viraemic infection by testing for HCVcAg – an HCV nucleocapsid peptide 22 (p22), which is released into the plasma during viral assembly and can be detected both early on and throughout the course of HCV infection *(269)*. Serological methods that test for detection of HCVcAg have the potential to be less costly and centralized than NAT, but evaluation has been limited in low-resource settings. There are now several assays commercially available for stand-alone detection of HCVcAg *(270)*. Detection of HCVcAg has also been used as an additional marker in a fourth-generation HCV Ag/Ab serological assay, because HCVcAg is detectable earlier than antibodies to HCV. However, the addition of core antigen was intended to increase sensitivity of the assay in early infection and not to differentiate seropositivity from active viraemic HCV infection.

11.3. Summary of the evidence

Two systematic reviews were undertaken, which evaluated the diagnostic accuracy for detection of viraemic HCV infection of (i) qualitative versus quantitative NAT *(see Web annex 5.7)*; and (ii) HCVcAg testing versus NAT (see Web annex 5.8) *(271)*.

Diagnostic accuracy and limit of detection of HCV NAT assays

The systematic review identified four eligible studies *(272–275)* that compared the performance of three quantitative HCV RNA NAT assays to a reference qualitative NAT (two assays used). Although early-generation qualitative NAT assays were able to detect the presence of HCV in plasma at concentrations a full log lower (i.e. about 10-fold less) than quantitative NAT assays, the lower limit of quantification of new versions of quantitative assays is now comparable to most commercial qualitative assays, i.e. 15 IU/mL.

Diagnostic accuracy and limits of detection of HCVcAg assays

There were 50 studies that evaluated seven commercial HCVcAg assays. There was significant variation in performance between the different assay brands (Table 11.1) *(271)*. The pooled sensitivity and specificity with 95% CI were: ARCHITECT 93.4% (95% CI: 88.7–96.2) and 98.7% (95% CI: 96.9–99.4); Ortho ELISA 93.2% (95% CI: 81.6–97.7) and 99.2% (95% CI: 87.9–100); and Hunan Jynda 59.5% (95% CI: 46–71.7) and 82.9% (95% CI: 58.6–94.3). The sensitivity for the Lumipulse was 95% (95% CI: 90.2– 99.8) in one study, but specificities could not be calculated. The estimates for the ARCHITECT assay were more homogeneous and precise as this assay has been the most extensively studied.

A pooled quantitative analysis of data available from three studies demonstrated a close correlation between HCVcAg and HCV RNA at viral loads above 3000 IU/mL.

The LoD for the most sensitive assay is 3 fmol/L HCVcAg or 0.06 pg/mL, which equates to an LoD of about ~1000–3000 IU/mL by NAT, and is consistent with the analytical sensitivity (LoD) reported by the manufacturer.

NAT assays are considered the reference standard for the detection of viraemia, but the quality of studies comparing quantitative versus qualitative assays for detection of viraemia was rated as low because of small numbers of studies and heterogeneity in populations.

The overall quality of the evidence for the recommendation to use HCVcAg was rated as low to moderate because of inconsistency and imprecision.

TABLE 11.1. Summary of diagnostic accuracy of HCV core antigen assays compared to NAT

Index test	Sample size (range)	Diagnostic accuracy (95% CI) Sensitivity	Diagnostic accuracy (95% CI) Specificity
Abbott Diagnostics GmbH, ARCHITECT HCV Ag Assay	20 (11–820)	93.4% (88.7–96.2)	98.7% (96.9–99.4)
Ortho-Clinical Diagnostics, Ortho ELISA-Ag	5 (1–177)	93.2% (81.6–97.7)	99.2% (87.9–99.9)
Bio-RAD Monolisa HCV Ag-Ab ULTRA	5 (525)	28.6–95%[a]	94.9% (89.9–99.8)[b]
EIKEN Lumispot HCV Ag	2 (235)	97.5–98.1%[a]	ND
Fujirebio Lumipulse Ortho HCV Ag	1 (80)	95% (90.2–99.8)[b]	ND
Hunan Jynda HCV Core Ag ELISA	4 (524)	59.5% (46–71.7)	82.9% (58.6–94.3)
DiaSorin S.A. Murex HCV Ag/Ab	4 (730)	50–100%[a]	83.8–100%[a]

CI: confidence interval; ND = no data.
[a] Meta-analysis not possible. Range of results seen across studies reported.
[b] Result from one study only.

11.4. Rationale for the recommendations
Balance of benefits and harms

Use of quantitative or qualitative NAT assays for detection of HCV RNA

The Guidelines Development Group made a strong recommendation for the use of a NAT assay (either qualitative or quantitative) as the preferred strategy for diagnosis of viraemic HCV infection based on moderate-/low-quality evidence for several reasons:

1. The new generation of quantitative and qualitative assays have the same LoD, which is around 15 IU/mL. However, quantitative assays are a reproducible method to detect and quantify HCV RNA in plasma or serum.

2. A supplementary review of the literature showed that that 95% of those with chronic infection have a viral load >10 000 IU/mL except, temporarily, a minority with partial viral control between 5 and 12 months post infection. Therefore, the range of clinically observed HCV viral loads is rarely below the lower range of the limit of quantification (LoQ) of quantitative assays, and most NAT assays (quantitative or qualitative) will capture the majority of viraemic infections.

3. Although quantitative RNA assays are considered the gold standard assays for the diagnosis and monitoring of HCV, the high cost of these assays and laboratory requirements means that they are not readily available in resource-limited settings. However, new NATs for use at or near the point of care for quantitation of HCV RNA are already available. These devices are easier to use than the laboratory-based NAT assays and can potentially improve access to diagnosis of viraemic HCV infection.

Use of HCV core antigen for detection of HCV RNA

The Guidelines Development Group recognized that there is limited access to NAT assays in resource-limited settings and that this represents an important barrier to antiviral treatment. The Group made a conditional recommendation to consider use of HCVcAg assays as an alternative to NAT to diagnose viraemic HCV infection, based on moderate-quality evidence, for several reasons:

1. HCVcAg assays can utilize existing serological testing platforms and are potentially lower-cost options than NAT. They could serve as a more affordable replacement to NAT for HCV detection in the future.

2. Although HCVcAg testing is currently limited to only a few platforms and even those with the highest performance do not reach the sensitivity of NAT, some well-performing HCVcAg assays have high sensitivity (up to 93.4% for certain commercial assays and high specificity (>98%), and good correlation with HCV RNA to an LoD of roughly 3000 IU/mL, which will detect over 95% of chronic HCV infections. However, it was noted that there was wide variation in sensitivity/specificity between assays and also within the same brand of assay for all but the Abbott ARCHITECT.

3. HCVcAg tests also offer the potential in the future to be applied as a one-step screening test as HCVcAg appears earlier than HCV antibodies (1–2 days after HCV RNA appears), has a high specificity, and so does not require any further confirmatory testing. However, such a strategy would be cost–effective only in very high-prevalence settings.

The risk in the use of HCVcAg is of potentially missing cases due to reduced clinical sensitivity. A further consideration is that it is preferable to select an assay that can be used for both diagnosis of viraemia and for test of cure to simplify the diagnostic pathway. On the basis of the limited current evidence, the HCVcAg assay cannot be recommended as a monitoring test.

Acceptability, values and preferences

The values and preferences survey identified preferences for future HCV testing strategies among respondents. Key preferences were for a single-step HCV diagnostic strategy with a low-cost point-of-care test for confirming viraemic infection (48% of respondents). Of these, 52% opted for an HCV RNA test because of its high sensitivity, and 35% for an HCVcAg assay because of its lower cost and ease of use. More than half the respondents were prepared to compromise on sensitivity down to 95% in order to gain a reduction in the price of the test. Forty-seven per cent of respondents also indicated a preference for a test that uses capillary blood and therefore could be more easily performed in point-of-care settings, even at the expense of test sensitivity. A short turnaround time (at least same day) was identified as another key consideration to reduce loss to follow up, cost of transportation, and enable providers to see more patients within a day.

Feasibility

The survey of hepatitis testing experience in 19 LMICs found that NAT for HCV RNA is available at a third of the sites but 40% of respondent countries do not have access to NAT for HCV diagnosis in their countries. The HCVcAg assay was not available at any site.

Resource considerations

The resources required for quantitative NAT were considered to be substantial, with the cost per test ranging from US$ 30 to US$ 200. Furthermore, the laboratory equipment is expensive and requires technicians with specialized training. The cost of testing for HCVcAg is currently US$ 25–50 (MSF data), which is comparable to qualitative NAT (US$ 43–51), but this is still a major barrier to its use.

11.5. Implementation considerations

1. Near patient or point-of-care (POC) technologies. The development of reliable and affordable POC NAT and HCVcAg tests able to diagnose viraemic infection in field settings will be crucial for expanding hepatitis testing services (*see* Chapter 17.3.5 – diagnostic innovations). These devices offer the possibility of a same-day diagnosis of viraemic infection either alone or when combined with an HCV antibody RDT and for test of cure. Since they are also more affordable than the laboratory-based assays, they can potentially improve access to early diagnosis, monitoring and linkage to care and treatment services, as well as reduce loss to follow up.

2. Immediate NAT directly after a positive serological result. The value of prompt testing for viraemia after a positive antibody result was highlighted, as patients with resolved HCV infection following spontaneous clearance can be reassured and those with viraemic infection could be promptly referred for care and treatment.

3. Genotyping. In most countries, there is a mix of HCV genotypes among persons with chronic HCV infection. The 2016 Hepatitis C treatment guidelines *(5)* provide recommendations on the preferred and alternative DAA regimens by HCV genotype. Therefore, knowing a patient's genotype is still important for determining the most appropriate treatment regimen. Genotype determination, however, is expensive and not available in all settings. Where genotype information is unavailable, pragmatic decision-making may be required, taking into account the common genotypes circulating in the affected population. However, as pangenotypic regimens become available over the next year, this will no longer be required.

Research gaps

- Establish the proportion of patients with chronic HCV infection with low viral loads that may be missed by HCV RNA or cAg assays that have a higher limit of detection (i.e. 3000 IU/mL).

- Evaluate the diagnostic accuracy, cost, cost–effectiveness and impact of HCVcAg or HCV RNA assays as a one-step diagnostic strategy.

- Assess the impact of HIV or HBV coinfection or genotype (particularly genotypes 4, 5 and 6, on which there are limited data) on detection of viraemia.

12. ASSESSMENT OF HCV TREATMENT RESPONSE - test of cure

12.1. Recommendation

Assessment of HCV treatment response	• Nucleic acid testing for qualitative or quantitative detection of HCV RNA should be used as test of cure at 12 or 24 weeks (i.e sustained virological response (SVR12 or SVR24)) after completion of antiviral treatment. *Conditional recommendation, moderate/low quality of evidence*

12.2. Background

Detection of HCV viraemia is important to assess the response to treatment *(276–278)*. Prior to the introduction of curative oral DAA treatment regimens, treatment with interferon (IFN)-based regimens required frequent monitoring of HCV viral load levels during therapy to decide whether treatment should be stopped, or treatment duration could be shortened. Previously, these multiple measurements included a viral load measurement at week 4 of therapy to help predict the efficacy of therapy, and then again at week 12 (early viral response, EVR), and finally at 12 and 24 weeks after completion of therapy to test for cure (sustained viral response, SVR).

These multiple assessments are now no longer relevant with the newer DAAs because of the relative infrequency of viral breakthrough and because the rate of viral load decline does not correlate with SVR. In fact, in most persons treated with DAAs, the viral load is undetectable 4 weeks after treatment initiation. In view of the high cost and relative unavailability of NAT testing for HCV RNA, this provides an important opportunity to reduce the frequency of on-treatment laboratory monitoring. HCVcAg testing has also been proposed as an alternative to HCV RNA for the diagnosis of viraemic HCV infection. However, there remains debate about whether HCVcAg can also be used as a tool for assessing the response to HCV antiviral treatment and to test for cure.

12.3. Summary of the evidence

The accuracy of HCVcAg for treatment monitoring and to confirm successful viral clearance (test of cure) was assessed by descriptive analysis of five studies *(279–283)* of two HCVcAg assays in comparison with HCV RNA NAT (qualitative and/or quantitative) (see *Web annex 5.8*). All studies were based on patients with mainly genotype 1b infection and on IFN-based therapy. The sensitivity of the HCVcAg assay in EVR ranged from 74% to 100% and specificity from 70% to 100%. SVR was assessed in only two studies with 100% sensitivity and specificity ranging from 94% to 100%. There were only three studies that evaluated the same assay – the Abbott ARCHITECT HCV Ag assay. There were no studies that evaluated the use of HCVcAg assay for monitoring treatment response using DAA IFN-free treatment regimens.

12.4. Rationale for the recommendation

Balance of benefits and harms

Use of qualitative or quantitative HCV RNA as a test of cure

The Guidelines Development Group recommended the use of either qualitative or quantitative NAT detection of HCV RNA as a test of cure at 12 weeks (or 24 weeks if 12 weeks is not possible) after completion of treatment. As shown in Chapter 11, these assays have a broad dynamic range from 12 to 7 700 000 IU/mL, and the reviews showed analytical sensitivity as low as 5 IU/mL for qualitative HCV RNA by NAT. Although either assay was recommended, the lower cost of qualitative assays for HCV RNA makes them preferable to quantitative NAT as a test of cure at 12 weeks *(284–287)*.

Use of HCVcAg as a test of cure

The Guidelines Development Group recognized that dependence on detection of HCV RNA by NAT to assess response to HCV antiviral treatment and test of cure, especially in remote settings, could be a barrier to the setting up of hepatitis C treatment and testing services. However, the data on HCVcAg in treatment monitoring and assessment of test of cure (SVR) was considered to be too limited to recommend its use as a substitute for HCV RNA.

Timing of test of cure

The Guidelines Development Group recognized that in the new era of treatment with curative DAA regimens, monitoring of viraemia during therapy with HCV RNA by NAT may no longer be necessary *(288)*, and that a single negative test of viral load at 12 weeks after completion of therapy (SVR12) is now the benchmark for assessing treatment outcome and cure used in all clinical studies of DAA-based regimens.

Acceptability, values and preferences

In the values and preferences survey of implementers and users of hepatitis testing services, almost half of the survey respondents expressed a preference for the test of cure to be performed 12 weeks after completion of HCV therapy because this was the earliest time point to reliably establish cure. However, one third expressed a preference for this to be performed more promptly after completion of treatment – at 4 weeks (20% of respondents) and 8 weeks (16%).

Feasibility

In the values and preferences survey, HCVcAg assay was reported as not available at any of the sites, and 40% of respondents also reported that they did not have access to HCV NAT in their countries.

Resource considerations

The availability of validated POC NAT assays, and further reduction in costs of both qualitative and quantitative NAT, will be critical to improve access to diagnosis and monitoring in LMICs.

12.5. Implementation considerations

1. **Re-infection.** The possibility of reinfection with HCV after successful treatment should be considered, and persons treated but who are still at active risk (e.g. current PWID) should be advised to retest annually for HCV RNA.

2. **Timing of test of cure.** A test of cure at 24 weeks (SVR24) after completion of treatment may be considered as an alternative SVR time-point, if SVR12 is not possible. Similarly, in populations for which there are limited data on the correlation between SVR12 and SVR24, e.g. patients with cirrhosis, HIV/HCV coinfection and other immunocompromised states, SVR24 may be considered.

3. **Impact of co-morbidities.** Clinical judgement based on the patient's clinical circumstances, such as presence of HIV coinfection, cirrhosis or renal impairment, potential drug interactions and clinical well-being during treatment, may necessitate more frequent monitoring for side-effects and disease progression.

Research gaps

- The impact of HIV or HBV coinfection and genotype on diagnostic accuracy of HCVcAg and quantitative/qualitative HCV RNA NAT as a test of cure should be assessed.
- The kinetics of HCVcAg with DAA treatment should be evaluated, and an optimal time-point identified to test for cure with DAA regimens using HCVcAg.
- The distribution of HCV viral load in the setting of viral rebound should be assessed to inform optimization of HCVcAg detection.
- Specific situations where quantitative NAT assay may be indicated, i.e. shortened DAA treatment course to 8 weeks, should be evaluated in those with lower baseline HCV RNA levels.
- The correlation between SVR12 and SVR24 should be evaluated in populations where there are more limited data, e.g. patients with cirrhosis, HIV/HCV coinfection and other immunocompromised states.

13. USE OF DRIED BLOOD SPOT SPECIMENS FOR SEROLOGICAL AND VIROLOGICAL TESTING

13.1. Recommendations

Topic	Recommendations
Serological testing	• The use of DBS specimens for HBsAg and HCV antibody serology testing[1] may be considered in settings where: - there are no facilities or expertise to take venous whole blood specimens; **or** - RDTs are not available or their use is not feasible; **or** - there are persons with poor venous access (e.g. in drug treatment programmes, prisons). *Conditional recommendation, moderate (HBV)/low (HCV) quality of evidence*
Detection of viraemia (nucleic acid testing)	• The use of DBS specimens to test for HBV DNA and HCV RNA for diagnosis of HBV and HCV viraemia[1], respectively, may be considered in settings where: - there is a lack of access to sites or nearby laboratory facilities for NAT, or provision for timely delivery of specimens to a laboratory; **or** - there are persons with poor venous access (e.g. in drug treatment programmes, prisons). *Conditional recommendation, low (HBV)/moderate (HCV) quality of evidence*

[1] Well-functioning laboratory specimens referral network and system for return of results should be in place to maximize the impact of DBS specimens. There are currently few assays where the manufacturer's instructions state that DBS specimens are validated for use. Therefore, currently use of DBS specimens would be considered "off-label".

13.2. Background

Significant scale up in access to hepatitis testing and treatment will require further simplification of the process of diagnosis and monitoring, and methods to facilitate access to testing, especially in decentralized settings, and among vulnerable populations worldwide, such as PWID and people in prison. DBS is an alternative specimen collection method that does not require venepuncture, and is being increasingly used to facilitate access to serological testing and NAT for HIV, hepatitis B and C, and other infectious diseases *(289–292)*, particularly in remote and underresourced regions with poor access to laboratory services, as well as for large epidemiological surveillance studies. DBS sampling involves obtaining a whole blood specimen, usually by capillary finger-stick (or heel-prick in infants), and embedding the drops of blood onto filter paper, or by pipetting venous blood onto filter paper. DBS specimens can then be transported from remote areas to a laboratory by standard means, e.g. posted to a laboratory, where testing would take place. The simplicity and relative ease of specimen collection, preparation, transport and storage make DBS specimens a potential option for serological testing and NAT in low-resource settings *(289)*.

An increasing number of studies have been undertaken to validate the use of DBS specimens to test for HBsAg and antibodies to HCV, and NAT for HBV DNA and HCV RNA *(291–293)*, including systematic reviews on HCV RNA detection using DBS specimens *(294)*, and on the uptake of HCV screening *(295)*.

13.3 Summary of the evidence

Four updated systematic reviews and meta-analyses were undertaken to evaluate the diagnostic accuracy and impact of using DBS specimens compared to venous blood specimens for hepatitis B and C serological testing and NAT *(see Web annex 5.9)*. The reviews evaluated the pooled sensitivity, specificity, positive and negative likelihood ratios, as well as the impact and duration of different storage conditions. Ten studies were included in the meta-analysis for HBsAg *(290, 293, 296–303)*, 17 studies for HCV antibody *(256, 293, 298, 299, 304–317)*, 10 studies for HBV DNA *(293, 301, 318–325)*, and 9 studies for HCV RNA *(305, 311, 312, 326–331)* based on an update of one study in an existing review *(294)*. The summary of results is shown in Table 13.1.

Serology

The pooled sensitivity for detection of HBsAg in DBS specimens compared to plasma or serum specimens was 92.9% (95% CI: 86.2–96.5%) and specificity 99.9% (95% CI: 96.2–99.7%), and for antibodies to HCV the sensitivity was 98% (95% CI: 94–99%) and specificity 99% (95% CI: 97–100%).

Impact of storage conditions. Most studies used storage conditions not applicable to typical field conditions (i.e. storage in a freezer or refrigerator). Those studies that investigated variation of results after storage of specimens in different conditions found that specimens could become false-positive with longer exposure at ambient temperatures for HCV antibody *(305, 326, 332)* and HBsAg *(302, 303)*.

Nucleic acid testing

Overall, studies and data were more limited for NAT than for serology testing, especially for HBV DNA, and had smaller sample sizes and were of lower quality. Nine studies contributed to the quantitative analysis of the diagnostic accuracy of HBV DNA measurement in DBS specimens compared to serum samples. Pooled sensitivity for HBV DNA measurement in DBS specimens was 96% (95% CI: 90–98%) and specificity 99% (95% CI: 55–100%), and for HCV RNA, 96.0% (95% CI: 93.4–97.6%) and 97.7% (95% CI: 94.7–99.0%). The descriptive review also shows a good correlation and strong association between quantitative values for HBV DNA on DBS specimens and in serum samples.

Impact of storage conditions. No study reported on storage conditions longer than 24 hours at room temperature for DBS specimens to test for HBV, but several studies that varied storage conditions for individual specimens found no effect on the qualitative result of these assays *(301, 323, 324)*. Several HCV RNA studies stored DBS specimens at ambient room temperature. While these storage conditions did not affect accuracy, and RNA positivity could still be detected with DBS specimens, quantitative signals decreased over time in two studies *(305, 332)*.

The quality of evidence for recommendations to use DBS for HBV and HCV serology was rated as low to moderate for HBV and low for HCV, and for HBV and HCV NAT, it was low for HBV and moderate for HCV.

Table 13.1. Summary of diagnostic performance of DBS specimens for serological and NAT testing

	DBS for HBsAg	DBS for anti-HCV	DBS for HBV DNA[1]	DBS for HCV RNA
No. of included studies	10 (SR), 9 (meta-anal)	18 (SR), 14 (meta-anal)	10 (SR), 9 (meta-anal)	9 (SR & meta-anal)
Total sample size	2481	4524	608	1250
Overall pooled sensitivity (95% CI)	92.9% [86.2–96.5]	98% [94–99]	96% [90–98]	96.0% [93.4–97.6]
Overall pooled specificity (95% CI)	99.0% [96.2–99.7]	99% [97–100]	99 [55–100]	97.7% [94.7–99.0]
Impact of storage	Cold chain: SN 78.7% [70–85] SP: 98.6% [68–100] ≥RT: SN: 96.1% [92–98] SP: 99.7% [98–100]	Storage at –20 °C associated with less variation compared to RT	Not possible to calculate because all accuracy studies conducted at –20 °C	Better result at –20 °C compared to RT; conflicting results re deterioration of sample at RT
Impact of duration of storage	Accuracy not affected if RT for ≤15 days (1 study) or 63 days (another study)	Accuracy not affected if RT for ≤3 days (1 study) or ≤6 days (another study) or ≤60 days (another study)	No effect on accuracy if 4–37 °C for ≤7 days (2 studies)	Conflicting results re deterioration over time

DBS: dried blood spot; meta-anal: meta-analysis; RT: room temperature; SN: sensitivity; SP specificity; SR: systematic review

[1] HBV DNA testing is not recommended for ruling out HBV infection if HBsAg is positive. HBV DNA detection can be used to explore occult HBV infection in persons testing negative for HBsAg. A large proportion of HBV-infected persons have a low HBV replication level (inactive carriers).

13.4. Rationale for the recommendations

Balance of benefits and harms

Benefits of use of DBS. (Table 13.2)

1. The Guidelines Development Group recognized that the principal benefit of DBS specimens is their potential to facilitate greater access to testing in settings where venepuncture and laboratory facilities are not easy to access. This is largely because of the relative ease of specimen collection with avoidance of venepuncture, easier handling that does not require high skill, transportation with a lower biohazard risk, and easier storage options.

2. The systematic reviews also showed generally high diagnostic accuracy of DBS specimens for both serology testing and NAT (although the evidence was more limited for evaluation of DBS for NAT, especially HBV DNA), and good precision based on low- to moderate-quality evidence. For HBsAg, sensitivity was 92.9% (range 86.2–96.5%), which is below the WHO prequalification standard for RDTs, and may lead to cases being missed.

3. Although data are still limited, DBS specimens are generally stable over time and maintain good accuracy in conditions with higher temperatures or humidity.

Risks of use of DBS. The Guidelines Development Group also recognized that several key caveats remain with the use of DBS specimens, as summarized in Table 13.2.

1. The main disadvantage is that the assay manufacturers have not yet validated their existing commercial assays with DBS specimens, which is required for regulatory approval for use of this specimen.

2. The minimum performance criteria of a DBS (whole blood) specimen for HBV and HCV serology and NAT are not well established.

3. Acceptable storage conditions need to be determined and validated by the manufacturer of the assay.

4. The evidence review was not able to support the use of certain commercial assays over others for DBS testing, or to suggest minimum performance criteria that should be retained for HBV and HCV screening on DBS specimens. There is also conflicting evidence on whether DBS increases the uptake of hepatitis testing among different vulnerable populations, as some studies have not confirmed this trend (*333–335*).

Overall, despite these caveats, the Guidelines Development Group considered that the procedural advantages make DBS specimens a good option for HBV and HCV testing in remote settings or specific populations. A conditional recommendation was therefore made to consider the use of DBS specimens as an option for both HBV and HCV serology and/or NAT, especially in specific settings, where there are either no facilities or expertise to take venous blood specimens, or there are persons with poor venous access (e.g. PWID and people in prisons). Use of DBS specimens for serological diagnosis was also recommended when RDTs are not available or their use is not feasible.

Assessing response to antiviral treatment
The Guidelines Development Group did not make a recommendation for the use of DBS specimens to assess response to antiviral treatment because of the lack of studies that have specifically addressed this question. Preliminary evidence shows that patients failing DAAs have high viral loads at 12 or 24 weeks after treatment completion, suggesting that testing with DBS may be feasible.

Limits of detection
For HBV DNA, existing WHO guidance *(6)* defines the HBV DNA threshold for initiation of treatment as ≥20 000 IU/mL, and does not recommend treating those with persistently normal ALT levels and low levels of HBV DNA replication (HBV DNA <2000 IU/mL) *(6)*. Therefore, assays for use in the field would not need to detect HBV DNA below 2000 IU/mL. Most individual studies suggest that the sensitivity of HBV DNA detection above 2000 IU/mL is good, and the LoD in DBS specimens is 900–4000 IU/mL, which means they would therefore be able to identify the majority of patients who require antiviral treatment.
For HCV RNA, it is estimated that the majority of people with viraemic HCV infection will have high viral loads >10 000 IU/mL. Although the thresholds at which HCV RNA can be detected using DBS specimens are not well characterized, the evidence suggests that qualitative detection of HCV RNA using DBS specimens is possible and accurate within this range.

Acceptability, values and preferences
The majority of respondents (implementers and users of hepatitis testing services) to the values and preferences survey from LMICs expressed a preference for DBS sampling because of the potential enhanced access to testing. They also considered that it was equally important for serology and NAT.

Feasibility and programmatic experience
There is limited programmatic experience with the use of DBS specimens for hepatitis B and C testing, but DBS has been incorporated into several screening programmes and has been used to scale up hepatitis C testing in certain populations in the UK *(336, 337)* and France *(338)*. It has also been used for testing of at-risk children for HBsAg at 12 months in the UK, and incorporated into research studies (*see* Box 13.1). These pilot programmes have already used DBS for antibodies to HCV on existing serological platforms without validation by the assay's manufacturer *(337, 339, 340)*.

Resource use
DBS sampling may reduce costs associated with sample collection, storage and transportation, potential for batch testing in a centralized laboratory, in addition to staff costs by facilitating task-shifting to lay workers.

Table 13.2. Summary of key benefits and challenges of DBS specimens

Benefits	Challenges and concerns
Ease of specimen collection. DBS specimen collection involves pricking a finger or a heel without the need for venepuncture, and so avoids the need for a trained health worker.	**Storage conditions.** Few studies have systematically examined the effects of storage and transport conditions on the accuracy of results from DBS specimens. However, some data suggest that there may be instability of results when stored for prolonged durations (more than 14 days) at high temperatures (room temperature and above) and humidity, particular for serological testing.
Ease of sample transport. Specimen transport and logistics are simplified as, apart from the advantage of avoiding venepuncture, DBS specimen handling does not require high skill and the biohazard risk is thought to be less (292).	**Manufacturers' validation.** Most manufacturers have not validated the use of their commercial assays with DBS specimens. In particular, procedures for pre-analytical treatment of specimens is not standardized, such as the type of filter paper, volume of capillary whole blood to be used, type of elution buffer and elution procedure. The impact on assay performance is uncertain but may result in potentially lower sensitivity/specificity.
Minimal training required. When DBS specimens are used for serological testing, the need for training in how to use and interpret RDTs is eliminated. Lay providers can be trained to take capillary whole blood samples without having to be trained in the use and reading of RDTs.	**Lack of assays with regulatory approval.** At present, there are few if any assays that have regulatory approval for the use of DBS as a specimen type for any HBsAg, anti-HCV, HBV DNA or HCV RNA assay.
Facility to allow multiplex testing. Multiplex testing of multiple diseases may be possible, such as HIV/HBV/HCV in combination using the same DBS specimen card. Both serological testing and NAT can be conducted from multiple spots on the same DBS card at the same laboratory, thereby avoiding the need for collecting a second sample from the patient.	**Assay cut-offs.** The use of a DBS specimen may require adjustment of the assay cut-off to determine test positivity for serological screening, as DBS specimens use a small volume of blood.
	Laboratory capacity. The actual laboratory work can be more difficult with a DBS specimen compared to a serum/plasma specimen, because it involves manual specimen processing, and requires a laboratory experienced in and competent at handling and processing these specimens. It also involves the need to maintain quality assurance of testing a specimen potentially off-label from the manufacturers' validated specimen types (293).

> **Box 13.1. Examples of programmatic use of DBS**
>
> - A voluntary counselling and testing service in France (The CheckPoint-Paris from the Kiosque) has offered rapid tests for screening and DBS for HCV RNA to confirm active infection since 2010. Hepatitis testing using DBS has also been adopted by associations such as the UK-based Hepatitis C Trust, le Réseau Hépatites LR in France, and by community pharmacists in the UK.
>
> - In 2012, the UK National Institute for Health and Care Excellence (NICE) recommended the use of DBS in certain settings for people with poor venous access and where there may be no facilities or expertise to take venous blood samples, such as prison and drug treatment services.
>
> - In France, guidelines from the Haute Autorité Sanitaire and AFEF-ANRS also recommended the use of DBS tests as an alternative to venous blood tests. However, the lack of standardization has limited the adoption of DBS, and as a result, there has been no clear recommendation for expansion of DBS testing.
>
> - In Scotland, 26% of new hepatitis C diagnoses during 2009–2013 were made in specialist drug services where DBS testing was introduced.
>
> - In a study of DBS sampling from substance misuse settings and prisons in Wales, less than 50% of those who were positive for anti-HCV returned for follow-up RNA testing, suggesting a low retention rate in care for those screened in such settings. Experience from DBS testing programmes in addiction centres in France has also observed a low rate of returning for results and linking to specialist care and treatment.

13.5. Implementation considerations

1. **Settings for DBS implementation.** The choice of whether to use DBS sampling for hepatitis B and C serological testing or NAT or both will depend on the health-care setting and infrastructure, and epidemiological context. Different programmes may opt for varying combinations: (i) DBS serology + DBS NAT (remote settings, hard-to-reach populations and those with poor venous access); (ii) RDT serology + DBS NAT (clinics, e.g. antenatal services); or (iii) EIA serology + plasma-based NAT (urban settings or larger hospitals). Therefore, if good-quality RDTs are available that can be performed using capillary blood, then the focus may be more on prioritizing DBS for NAT testing of HBV DNA and HCV RNA. However, if RDTs are not available and there are no facilities or expertise to take venous blood samples, then DBS testing may be equally important to increase access to serological testing as well as NAT and, conveniently, both could be performed from the same specimen if multiple spots are taken. Use of DBS may also be useful when large numbers of individuals are being tested at the same point in time, e.g.

drug treatment centres, prisons, or where polyvalent screening for multiple diseases, such as HIV/HBV/HCV, is being undertaken, but where multiplex RDTs for this purpose are not available or are more costly *(298)*.

2. **Validation of DBS with manufacturers' assays.** The use of DBS specimens has not yet been validated by assay manufacturers with their commercial assays, and under different storage and transport conditions. Addressing this is a priority for implementation, together with access to appropriate laboratory facilities and experience.

3. **Laboratory QA/QC.** The adoption of DBS sampling in a hepatitis testing programme requires the availability of a centralized laboratory experienced in and competent at handling and processing this sample type, as well as maintaining QA of testing a specimen potentially off-label from the manufacturers' validated specimen types.

4. **Training.** Lay workers will need to be trained to perform finger-prick DBS, and systems put in place for timely and efficient communication of results.

5. **Reducing loss to follow up.** The mobility and instability of some vulnerable populations has raised concerns that DBS may be associated with a low rate of returning for results and linkage to care and treatment. This is suggested by reports of low rate of return and linkage to care and treatment in drug treatment programme centres in France, particularly with DBS testing.

Research gaps

A major constraint to implementation of DBS sampling is the limited programmatic experience with its use for hepatitis testing in different settings. Priority areas for research and development include development of manufacturers' guidance and regulatory approval of commercial assays using DBS specimens, and the establishment of large-scale demonstration projects of DBS for hepatitis serological testing and NAT in different settings.

Specific research areas include the following:

- Larger diagnostic accuracy and validation studies should be conducted on the use of DBS specimens for serology and NAT with optimal assay cut-offs, and across a range of storage and transport conditions common in the field (i.e. no cold chain, high and low humidity). This should also include additional studies in HIV-coinfected patients.

- The optimal preparation of DBS specimens prior to analysis should be studied. This includes differences between capillary versus venous blood, most appropriate volume of capillary whole blood and best type of filter paper to be used.

- The use of DBS should be validated for monitoring of treatment response and HCV test of cure (SVR at 12 or 24 weeks) post DAA therapy, including threshold for detection. This includes validation of the rate of degradation of HCV RNA and detectability when stored at ambient temperatures and high humidity for different time periods.

- The diagnostic performance and impact on linkage to care of one DBS specimen card for serology and NAT should be compared with POC HCV RNA NAT or HCVcAg technologies in different settings, including mobile and outreach testing programmes and in prisons.

14. IMPROVING THE UPTAKE OF TESTING AND LINKAGE TO CARE AND PREVENTION

14.1. Recommendations

Topic	Recommendations
Uptake of testing and linkage to care	• All facility- and community-based hepatitis testing services should adopt and implement strategies to enhance uptake of testing and linkage to care. *Strong recommendation, moderate quality of evidence* • The following evidence-based interventions should be considered to promote uptake of hepatitis testing and linkage to care and treatment initiation: *(Conditional recommendations)* - **Peer and lay health worker support in community-based settings** *(moderate quality of evidence).* - **Clinician reminders** to prompt provider-initiated, facility-based HBV and HCV testing in settings that have electronic records or analogous reminder systems *(very low quality of evidence).* - **Provision of hepatitis testing as part of integrated services** within mental health/substance use services *(very low quality of evidence).*

14.2. Background

Uptake of testing and linkage to care are both essential initial components of the hepatitis B and C care continuum (Fig. 1.1). However, currently, levels of uptake of testing for hepatitis B and C are very low *(341, 342)*, and a large proportion of people living with viral hepatitis B and C are unaware of their infection, especially in LMICs, and those from vulnerable populations, such as PWID, sex workers or migrants. Poor linkage to care and loss to follow up after receiving a diagnosis of hepatitis B or C is a further challenge, contributing to delayed treatment initiation. Population-level data on the care continuum for viral hepatitis is limited, but even in high-income countries, only a small fraction of the estimated population living with HBV or HCV is ultimately treated and achieves viral suppression *(341, 342)*. Those who test negative, if at continuing high risk, as well as those who test positive, need linkage to prevention services and HBV vaccination. Without linkage to prevention, treatment and care, testing and learning one's hepatitis B or C status has limited value. Suboptimal linkage to prevention, care and treatment results in avoidable morbidity and mortality, poorer treatment outcomes, increased cost of care, and preventable transmission

Multiple factors may hinder the successful uptake of testing and linkage to care and prevention. These include patient-level factors (such as depression, lack of social or family support, and fear of disclosure), as well as structural or economic factors such as stigma and discrimination, distance from care sites, lack of or cost of transportation, and long waiting times at the facility) *(343)*. Hepatitis C also disproportionally affects individuals with comorbid mental health or substance use issues. Traditionally, services for hepatitis, mental health and substance use have been provided by separate clinicians or teams often located in different health facilities, which may contribute to HCV treatment dropout and/or treatment failure *(344)*.

Optimizing the impact of effective treatments and prevention will require interventions to both expand uptake of testing and improve linkage to care and retention across the care continuum, from initial screening to treatment initiation and viral suppression (HBV) or cure (HCV). Such interventions may vary based on the local context, including the health-care delivery system, geography and target population. There are several well-established evidence-based interventions that improve linkage to care and treatment of people who have received an HIV-positive diagnosis, and were included as recommendations in the WHO 2015 *HIV consolidated testing guidelines (11)* and the 2016 *ARV consolidated guidelines (23)*, which may also apply to viral hepatitis care and prevention.

14.3. Summary of the evidence

A systematic review was undertaken to assess the impact of different interventions to enhance five key steps along the continuum of care for chronic viral hepatitis – screening, linkage to care, treatment uptake, treatment adherence, and ultimately viral suppression. Fifty-four studies were included in the review, of which 37 studies addressed interventions and outcomes across the HCV care continuum, 15 across the HBV care continuum, and two across both *(334, 345–397)* (see *Web annex 5.11*) *(398)*. Thirty-three studies were included in a meta-analysis that generated pooled effect size estimates for different outcomes. Interventions to improve retention along the HBV continuum of care were limited to promoting testing and linkage to care, while interventions along the HCV continuum of care addressed all five steps. Interventions to address adherence, viral suppression, and uptake of HCV testing were the best studied, but there were few methodologically rigorous studies for promoting linkage to care, and particularly few studies on HBV. All studies except one *(370)* were from high-income countries. Most existing studies were rated as being of low or very low methodological quality, because of risk of bias due to study design issues, and a high degree of heterogeneity across studies.

Promotion of HBV testing by lay health workers

Nearly half (7/15) of the interventions to improve the uptake of HBV testing involved lay health worker interventions *(348, 354, 368, 376, 388–390)*. The majority of these were one-time activities that delivered educational content tailored to a particular community's cultural and social context, mainly Asian communities in the United States or Canada. Pooled meta-analysis from six studies showed that a single HBV test promotion intervention by lay health workers increased HBV testing rates compared to groups that received no or unrelated educational interventions (relative risk [RR] = 2.68 [1.82–3.93]). The quality of evidence was rated as moderate.

Clinician reminders to prompt HCV testing during clinical visits

Unlike interventions to improve HBV testing, which were primarily delivered in community settings, all 11 of the interventions to improve HCV testing either targeted health-care providers or took place at established health-care facilities *(333, 334, 358, 360, 362, 363, 371, 374, 379, 385, 386)*. Providers were prompted by reminders to either order HCV tests if patients belonged to a high-risk birth cohort *(371)*, reported risk behaviour *(360)* or both *(374)*, using reminder stickers attached to patient charts or in an electronic medical records system *(371)*. These studies found that clinician reminders to prompt HCV screening during clinical visits substantially increased HCV testing rates compared to no clinician reminders (RR = 3.70 [95% CI: 1.81–7.57]). The quality of evidence was rated as very low.

Integrated care between mental health and HCV treatment specialists

Several studies evaluated interventions providing "coordinated", "integrated", or "multidisciplinary" care to improve treatment adherence and viral suppression in patients with mental health issues. *(345, 352, 359, 365, 369, 381)*. Three RCTs demonstrated that interventions facilitating referral and scheduling to specialist sites increased patient attendance at HCV specialist visits (RR = 1.57 [95% CI: 1.03–2.41], moderate-quality evidence). Individually tailored mental health counselling and motivational therapy to treat mental health and/or substance use issues also increased the number of patients who were regarded as eligible for treatment compared to usual care (OR = 3.43, 95% CI: 1.81–6.49). Coordinated care between mental health and treatment specialists along with psychological therapy and counselling for patients with mental health and/or substance use comorbidities increased HCV treatment initiation (OR = 3.03 [95% CI: 1.24–7.37]), improved treatment completion (RR = 1.22 [95% CI: 1.05–1.41]), and increased SVR (RR = 1.21 [95% CI: 1.07–1.38]) compared to usual care. Nurse-led therapeutic educational interventions also improved treatment completion and increased SVR). The quality of evidence was rated as low to very low.

Interventions to promote linkage to care for HIV

There are several well-established evidence-based interventions that improve linkage to care and treatment of people who have received an HIV-positive diagnosis, and were included as recommendations in the WHO 2015 *HIV consolidated guidelines on HIV testing services (11)* and the 2016 *ARV consolidated guidelines (23)*. Box 14.1 outlines some of these approaches, which may also be applicable to viral hepatitis care and prevention.

Box 14.1. Good practices for promoting linkage to care from HIV testing services

- Comprehensive home-based testing, which includes offering home assessment and home-based treatment initiation;
- Integrated services, where testing, prevention, treatment and care, TB and STI screening, and other relevant services are provided together at a single facility or site;
- Providing on-site or immediate testing with same-day results;
- Providing assistance with transport, such as transportation vouchers, if the treatment site is far from the testing service site;
- Decentralized treatment provision and community-based distribution of treatment;
- Support and involvement of trained lay providers who are peers and act as peer navigators, expert patients/clients, and community outreach workers to provide support, and identify and reach people lost to follow up;
- Intensified post-test counselling by community health workers;
- Using communication technologies, such as mobile phones and text messaging, which may help with disclosure, adherence and retention;
- Providing brief strengths-based case management, which emphasizes people's self-determination and strengths, is client-led and focuses on future outcomes, helps clients set and accomplish goals, establishes good working relationships among the client, health worker and other sources of support in the community, and provides services outside of office settings;
- Promoting partner testing may increase rates of testing and linkage to care.

Source: Consolidated guidelines on HIV testing services. Geneva: WHO; 2015 *(11).*

14.4. Rationale for the recommendations

Balance of benefits and harms

The Guidelines Development Group recognized that poor uptake of viral hepatitis testing and linkage to care is a major barrier to access to care and treatment. To expand access to testing and treatment, programmes need to not only make use of multiple testing approaches at the facility and community levels, but also adopt interventions to promote optimal linkage to prevention and treatment. The Guidelines Development Group made a strong recommendation for the general adoption and implementation of a series of relatively simple, low-cost but effective strategies (promotion of testing by lay health workers, clinician reminders and coordinated care between hepatitis and mental health specialists) to enhance uptake of hepatitis testing and linkage to care, based on generally low-quality evidence from the systematic review.

Specifically, promotion of HBV screening activities by lay health workers increased HBV testing uptake, while clinician reminders to prompt HCV screening during clinical visits increased HCV testing rates. Coordinated care between hepatitis and mental health specialists along with psychological therapy and counselling for patients with mental health and/or substance use comorbidities also increased HCV treatment initiation and treatment completion, and resulted in higher SVR rates. Integration of services among certain populations of individuals with HCV such as PWID may also be useful. The Guidelines Development Group also considered evidence from recent systematic reviews on interventions to improve linkage to care following HIV testing, which was considered relevant to hepatitis care and treatment services.

Feasibility, acceptability, and resource use

Education and support for peer and lay health-care workers. The findings are also consistent with the growing body of evidence demonstrating that lay health workers effectively perform a range of interventions that would otherwise be undertaken by trained medical personnel, strengthen service delivery capacity in a variety of clinical settings in LMICs *(399–402)*, and are critical to supporting decentralization of services and non-facility-based testing. Evidence supports such peer-led interventions as being feasible and acceptable to both those individuals screened and lay health workers themselves *(403)*. The low-cost nature of this intervention could facilitate its use in resource-limited settings. The lay health workers in the seven studies received training in order to help tailor the educational intervention; this training component was relatively simple and of low cost.

Clinician reminders. Clinician reminders are consistent with the broader shift towards standardizing clinical practice, including provider-initiated screening and systems-based approaches to improving clinical outcomes. Implementation is relatively easy and similar systems have demonstrated effectiveness in multiple disease modalities, such as breast *(404)* and colorectal cancer screening *(405)*.

Integrated care. Integrating HCV screening and treatment with mental health and substance use services is feasible and acceptable to targeted clients *(195, 406)*. Chapter 17 on service delivery provides a range of examples of integrated care in different settings promoting linkage to hepatitis care. While the interventions addressing multidisciplinary or integrated care in the evidence review were diverse, a likely key contributor to improved outcomes was co-location and coordination of services.

Costs and cost–effectiveness

None of the studies identified in the systematic review reported estimates of the direct cost or cost–effectiveness of interventions. However, effective linkage to hepatitis care and treatment following a positive diagnosis would be expected to improve programme effectiveness, support earlier treatment initiation and reduce loss to follow up before treatment initiation, thus resulting in potential cost savings along the continuum of care.

14.5. Implementation considerations

1. **Policies on linkage to care.** Proactive linkage approaches are a critical component of comprehensive hepatitis testing services. Countries should ensure that they have specific policies and strategies to improve and prioritize linkages between hepatitis testing and prevention, treatment and care services. Interventions that impact on multiple steps along the care continuum will generally be more resource efficient. The effectiveness of linkage will vary for different testing approaches.

2. **Linkage to prevention services.** As for HIV *(11)*, a range of prevention services should be available for those diagnosed with hepatitis, as well as for those who test negative. Linkage to prevention services for people who test HBV or HCV negative is not well documented or studied. Supporting linkage to prevention services is particularly important for those with high ongoing risk, such as PWID and serodiscordant couples.

3. **Monitoring and evaluation**. Monitoring people's linkage following hepatitis testing is critical to strengthening the treatment and prevention cascades. The success of linkage should be measured by enrolment in care and not by intermediary process indicators such as the number of referrals issued, and areas identified for improvement. Without strategies that ensure linkage and enrolment in care, the effect of hepatitis testing in reducing HBV or HCV transmission, morbidity and mortality cannot be fully realized.

Research gaps

Most existing studies were rated as being of low or very low methodological quality, and there has been a lack of methodologically rigorous studies, in particular, on interventions to promote uptake of HBV and HCV testing, linkage to HBV treatment uptake, and HCV treatment in the era of DAA therapy. There is a need for studies evaluating the effectiveness, costs and cost–effectiveness of packages of different interventions and combinations of interventions to optimize engagement and retention, and treatment outcomes for people living with HBV and HCV along the continuum of care, especially in LMICs.

PART 3: IMPLEMENTATION

Laboratory testing:
- How to organize laboratory testing services for viral hepatitis

Service delivery:
- Pre- and post-test counselling
- Service delivery approaches to hepatitis testing
- Testing issues in priority populations
- Strategic planning for implementing testing services and approaches

15. IMPLEMENTING LABORATORY TESTING SERVICES FOR VIRAL HEPATITIS

15.1. Key elements for national testing services

The efficient coordination of testing services at the national level is important for an effective and sustainable national hepatitis testing programme. Table 15.1 summarizes the key elements for countries to consider while planning or further expanding testing for viral hepatitis[4] to ensure the quality and accuracy of testing.

Table 15.1. Key elements to consider while planning and expanding hepatitis testing services

Section 15.2	National framework for viral hepatitis testing	National testing policy
		National hepatitis strategic plan (including testing)
		National regulatory mechanisms (for diagnostic products, staff and services)
		National reference laboratory
Section 15.3	Building capacity for testing services	Human resource management
		Inventory management (procurement and supply chain)
		Storage and transportation
		Equipment management
		Laboratory information management systems
Section 15.4	Product selection	Monitoring testing algorithms
		Post-marketing surveillance of diagnostics
Section 15.5	Assuring the quality of testing services	Quality management system
		Quality control
		Personnel and training
Section 15.6	Assuring the safety of testing services	Facilities and safety

Adapted from Asia Pacific strategy for strengthening health laboratory services (2010–2015). Manila/Delhi: WHO; 2010 (http://www.searo.who.int/about/administration_structure/cds/BCT_Asia_Pacific_Strategy10-15.pdf, accessed 06 February 2017). Development of national health laboratory policy and plan. Manila/Delhi: WHO; 2011 (http://www.wpro.who.int/health_technology/documents/docs/Nationalhealthlab2_0F38.pdf?ua=1, accessed 06 February 2017).

A national technical working group should be developed to discuss and agree on each of the different laboratory aspects. It should comprise representatives from patient groups and civil society, public and private testing providers, national governmental agencies (national regulatory authorities, directorate of laboratory services, viral hepatitis programmes), laboratory specialists, programme experts, other implementing partners and nongovernmental agencies.

15.2. National framework for viral hepatitis testing

A framework approach is useful for guiding national authorities on how to arrange testing services that allow access to all populations that would benefit most from testing and linkage to prevention and antiviral treatment.

15.2.1. National hepatitis testing policy

A national testing policy for viral hepatitis is a statement of intent to provide testing services for viral hepatitis. It should set out the goals and objectives of the national testing services and define who is responsible for testing services at each level of the tiered testing network (*see* Fig. 15.2). It should be complementary to the wider national health policy, with a link to the justice system, given that many key populations at risk of acquiring viral hepatitis live in prisons and other closed settings. The national testing policy may be used to engage and build consensus through active participation with stakeholders for its development. This allows for all implementing partners to understand the national priorities for testing in all settings to reach equity in testing coverage. This document will contribute to the development of a national strategic plan for viral hepatitis that includes testing.

15.2.2. National hepatitis strategic plans (including testing)

A national strategic plan for viral hepatitis *(16)* that includes testing should describe how practically testing services will be established and delivered to support different testing objectives, i.e. diagnosis, prevention, surveillance and treatment. It allows for planning of public and private testing services in the context of the different tiers of the testing network (level 0 through to level 4; *see* Fig. 15.2). Development of national and regional plans should include all relevant stakeholders involved in organizing the structure and network of facilities for hepatitis testing.

Strategic planning for testing services requires first a situation analysis (or needs assessment) to identify and map all existing facilities (public and private; facility- and community-based) that have the capacity to undertake viral hepatitis testing, with an assessment of their organizational structure, infrastructure, technical and human resources, and financing. A minimum package of testing services to be provided at each of the four levels of the health-care system (*see* Fig. 15.2), as well as at the community level, should be agreed upon and articulated in the plan. Each testing facility will require a specific and sufficient budget, a suitable infrastructure, with some facilities requiring additional infrastructure (such as reliable water and equipment). Plans should also include a monitoring and evaluation mechanism, with a baseline, targets and indicators in order to measure progress and impact.

15.2.3. National regulatory mechanisms (for diagnostics, staff and services)

Each national programme should ensure that there are regulatory mechanisms that can perform oversight functions for the various activities of the viral hepatitis testing programme. These may be carried out by the health authority and health product regulatory authorities or through a designated governmental agency. The scope of regulation should encompass regulatory controls (pre-market and post-market) for IVDs available for sale and use within the country, certification of competency of testing staff, and accreditation of testing services. An effective oversight system gives confidence in the testing services to all stakeholders.

For countries that do not currently possess capacity and/or competency to regulate IVDs and other laboratory equipment and items, the WHO prequalification assessment serves as a mechanism to provide an independent assessment of the quality, safety and performance of IVDs that are intended for sale and use in resource-limited settings. A number of guidance documents are available to direct nascent regulators in their capacity-building efforts.

WHO conducts the prequalification assessment of IVDs using a standardized procedure to determine if the product meets WHO prequalification requirements. The assessment consists of three key components:

- review of the safety, quality and performance of the assay presented in a **product dossier** prepared by the manufacturer;
- desk review of the quality management systems applied during production, followed by a **site inspection;**
- independent **performance evaluation** of performance and operational characteristics.

15.2.4. National reference laboratory for oversight

At least one laboratory with the relevant expertise and experience could be designated as a national reference laboratory for viral hepatitis (level 4; *see* Fig. 15.2). A national public health or disease-specific reference laboratory is generally suitable for this task.

The role of the reference laboratory may include:
- provision of QC specimens;
- organization of quality assessment schemes;
- training and supervisory support.

15.3. Building capacity for testing services

Building or expanding existing capacity for viral hepatitis testing services should be considered in the wider framework of expanding access to testing services for a range of related diseases. The rise in use of multi-disease platforms for testing and the need to service coinfected individuals (such as HIV/HCV-coinfected patients) means that development of a trained and motivated health workforce should be considered across disease control programmes.

15.3.1. Human resource management

A range of personnel may be required for the different roles in testing services, including phlebotomists, test operators (laboratory technicians, POC test providers), data clerks and other auxiliary staff. The national strategic plan should detail how testing staff will be trained and certified, with their roles and responsibilities made clear. All staff should have appropriate qualifications, such as certifications according to national guidelines, and demonstrated proficiency in performing the tasks within their scope of work. Supervisory support to staff and regular site visits as part of a quality assessment system provides an opportunity for troubleshooting and feedback to higher management.

15.3.2. Inventory management (procurement and supply chain of assays and reagents)

Continuity in the supply of test kits, reagents and other consumables required for testing depends on reliable and responsive procurement and supply systems. Stock-outs of test kits or essential consumables can contribute to poor testing services. The testing programme should ensure that procurement procedures (either through a centralized medical store or direct from the supplier) are conducted in accordance with best global practice for procurement. Importantly, any bidding or evaluation of bidding should be conducted in a fair and transparent manner.

To support inventory management, testing services at user level should have appropriate systems in place to monitor stocks and expiry dates of test kits and reagents, as well a method to track consumption and wastage.

> **Further reading**
>
> Forthcoming second edition of Guidance for procurement of in vitro diagnostics and related laboratory items and equipment. Geneva: WHO; 2013. First edition available on the WHO website (http://www.who.int/diagnostics_laboratory/procurement/131024_procurement_of_diagnostics_finalversion.pdf?ua=1, accessed 06 February 2017).

15.3.3. Storage and transportation

All test kits and reagents should be transported and stored under controlled conditions, according the manufacturer's instructions for use of the product. Testing services should ensure that so-called room temperature-stable test kits such as RDTs are stored according to their labelling.

15.3.4. Equipment management

When purchasing diagnostics that require instrumentation, such as analysers (either closed or open platform, polyvalent or otherwise), ancillary equipment (e.g. refrigerator, freezer, incubators), and other equipment that requires installation and validation (e.g. autoclaves, water purification systems), it is necessary to ensure that these are maintained. This means calibration upon installation, as well as preventive and corrective maintenance, which should be foreseen as part of financial planning and procurement procedures.

> **Further reading**
>
> Maintenance manual for laboratory equipment, 2nd edition. Geneva: WHO; 2008 (http://apps.who.int/iris/bitstream/10665/43835/2/9789241596350_eng_low.pdf, accessed 06 February 2017).

15.3.5. Laboratory information management systems

Information management consists of paper-based and electronic systems for storing records and documents, including laboratory information management systems and mobile mechanisms that provide testing results or reminders to health-care facility staff or clients. It is closely linked to documentation and record-keeping.

To assure the quality and integrity of the test status given to a client, the testing service must minimize the risk of transcription errors. Assigning patient identification numbers and specimen identification numbers to each subsequent specimen received from the same individual will serve to reduce the possibility of transcription errors. It will also protect the confidentiality of people undergoing testing.

15.4 Product selection

While a testing strategy provides a generic approach to how many assays should be used and how many tests should be conducted on each assay, a testing algorithm defines the specific products (assay by brand name) to be used in a given testing strategy. The design of a testing algorithm will be determined by the specific disease marker to be tested for, and operational aspects such as the required expertise of the users, infrastructure and testing conditions, and assay characteristics. Selection should include some consideration of products that have been approved by (i.e. conforms to requirements of) stringent regulatory assessment, such as by the WHO prequalification programme or any of the founding members of the Global Harmonization Task Force (GHTF)[5] (Table 15.2).

---

[5] Founding members of the Global Harmonization Task Force are Australia, Canada, European Union, Japan, USA.

TABLE 15.2. Examples of stringent regulatory assessments

Regulatory jurisdiction	Risk class	Documentary evidence
WHO prequalification	All classes	WHO prequalification public report
European Union	Annex II, List A	EC Full Quality Assurance Certificate
		EC Production Quality Assurance Certificate
		EC Type-Examination Certificate
US Food and Drug Administration	Class III	PMA letter or BLA license
Health Canada	Class IV	Medical Device Licence and summary report for a Class IV IVD
		CMDCAS-issued ISO 13485 Certificate
Therapeutic Goods Administration (TGA), Australia	Class 4	TGA Licence for Manufacture
		TGA Issued ISO 13485 Certificate
		AUST R Number
		TGA Full Quality Assurance Certificate
		TGA Type-Examination Certificate
		TGA Production Quality Assurance Certificate
Japan Ministry of Health, Labour and Welfare (JMHLW)	Class III	JMHLW Minister's Approval
		JMHLW License for Manufacturer
		JMHLW Recognised Foreign Manufacturer

BLA: Biologics License Application; CMDCAS: Canadian Medical Devices Conformity Assessment System; EC: European Commission; PMA: pre-market approval

If there are no products available that meet these quality criteria (WHO prequalified or stringent review by GHTF founding member), then efforts should be made to review any other existing quality certification held by the manufacturer for the product of intended supply. This might include a request from the supplier to provide

- a list of all quality reviews conducted on the product;
- all internationally recognized standards such as ISO 13485 or equivalent.

The performance of potential candidate assays may have been published as independent performance evaluations in the peer-reviewed literature. The Standards for Reporting Diagnostic Accuracy (STARD) criteria should be used to exclude low-quality studies *(407)*.

15.4.1. Monitoring testing algorithms

A periodic assessment of the programmatic performance of diagnostics should be conducted. For example, when testing for HCV, if there are low rates of HCV viraemia in those that are HCV-antibody seropositive, this might indicate that there are high rates of false-positive results (poor specificity) for the serological assay(s). Conversely, if seroprevalence rates are low but a higher proportion are found to have detectable HCV RNA, then the possibility of false-negative results should be considered. Either scenario should trigger further revalidation of the testing algorithm to facilitate the selection of assays with increased sensitivity and/or specificity.

The following quality indicators should be monitored, as appropriate:

- rate of defective consumables, e.g. specimen transfer pipettes, lancets;
- rate of invalid test devices (if single-use devices such as RDTs);
- rate of invalid runs (disaggregated by error codes);
- rate of equipment breakdown and respective down-time rate of out-of-range QC results; and
- rate of discrepant results within a testing algorithm consisting of two or more assays.

15.4.2. Post-market surveillance of diagnostics

Once a product is placed on the market, its quality, safety and performance must be monitored to ensure that diagnostics continue to meet standards. WHO has established a system for post-market surveillance of diagnostics that supplements the obligations of manufacturers, who must also conduct their own post-market evaluation activities.

In this context, post-market surveillance consists of the following:

- **proactive post-market surveillance** (to identify any problem before use) through in-country lot verification testing, both before and after distribution of test kits to testing sites; and

- **reactive post-market surveillance** (when a problem has been identified during the use of the diagnostic) through reporting and evaluation of complaints, including reports of adverse events, and any required actions to correct the problem and prevent recurrence.

Lot verification testing conducted independently of the manufacturer is particularly useful where manufacturing quality has not been adequately assured, and to verify that an assay has minimal lot-to-lot variation *(408)*.

15.5. Assuring the quality of testing services

15.5.1. Quality management systems, irrespective of the testing setting

Effective quality management systems are essential for the overall effectiveness of a hepatitis testing programme. It should encompass all activities of the testing programme and not be limited to laboratories only, but include testing in health- and community-based facilities.

Any site conducting hepatitis testing should implement a quality management system that incorporates the 12 interconnected components summarized in Fig. 15.1. Many of these components have already been described in the context of the national framework for organizing testing services for viral hepatitis *(409)*.

FIG. 15.1. The 12 components of quality management systems

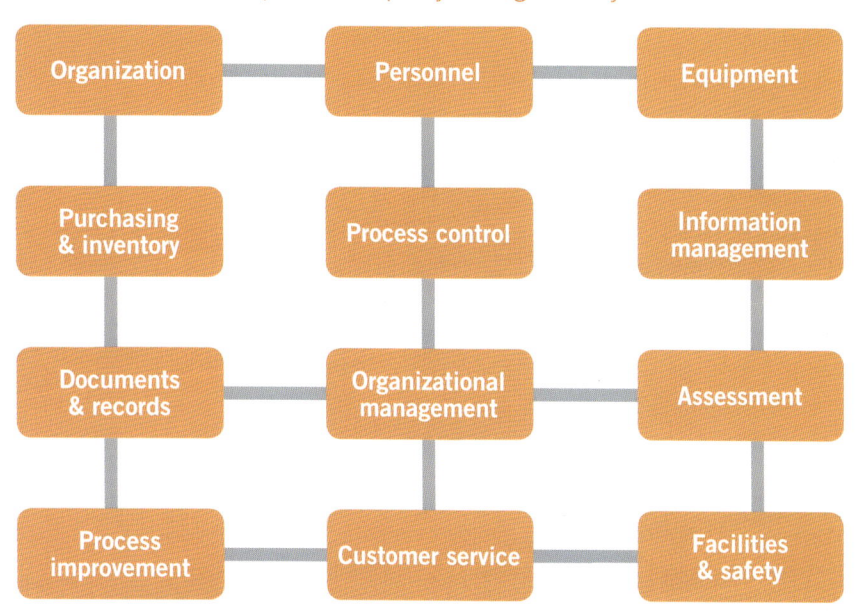

Organization	Personnel	Equipment
Purchasing & inventory	Process control	Information management
Documents & records	Organizational management	Assessment
Process improvement	Customer service	Facilities & safety

Source: Laboratory quality management system: handbook. Geneva: WHO: 2011 (http://www.who.int/ihr/publications/lqms/en/, accessed 06 February 2017).

> **Further reading**
>
> Laboratory quality management system: handbook. Geneva: World Health Organization; 2011 (http://www.who.int/ihr/publications/lqms/en/, accessed 06 February 2017).
>
> Improving the quality of HIV-related point-of-care testing: ensuring reliability and accuracy of test results. Geneva: World Health Organization; 2015 (http://www.who.int/hiv/pub/toolkits/handbook-point-of-care-testing/en/, accessed 06 February 2017).

Quality assurance (QA) should be seen as an integral part of the continuing roles and responsibilities of each and every staff member. Through this QA framework, countries can plan, implement, evaluate, improve and sustain QA activities. Such frameworks and provisions apply not only to test accuracy but also to ensuring the quality of pre-test information and post-test counselling.

15.5.2. Quality control

Quality control (QC), also known as process control, refers to processes and activities to ensure that testing procedures are performed correctly, that environmental conditions are suitable and that the assay works as expected. The intention of QC is to detect, evaluate and correct errors due to assay failure, environmental conditions or operator performance before results are reported. Hence, QC is a multistep process with certain checkpoints throughout the testing process.

Before testing (pre-analytical)
- Ensure the appropriate sample type and/or volume has been used.
- Check the expiry of test kits and required consumables.

While testing (analytical)
- Ensure that any QC specimens have been run (e.g. test kit controls and/or external QC specimen) and that the results are within QC acceptance criteria.
- Ensure that a test result is read correctly.

After testing (post-analytical)
- Double-check the report of test status to the client.

Internal QC refers to processes within the assay that check whether the test procedure is working; the appearance of a control line for HBsAg or anti-HCV RDTs is an example of internal QC.

As an addition to the test kit controls, **external quality control specimens** may be produced. These are prepared and validated for the assay by the specimen provider, usually the national reference laboratory or commercial entity, separately from the manufacturer. Many errors occur due to incorrect transcription of testing results and reporting of the status. All necessary steps should be taken to mitigate these errors such as rechecking the reports and re-reading visually read assays independently by a second individual *(409)*.

15.5.3. Personnel and training

All testing services must employ an adequate number of trained, certified and supported personnel to conduct each of the elements of hepatitis B and C testing for the expected number of tests conducted and the number of people being served. To assess and manage human resource planning, tools such as the WHO *Workload indicators for staffing need* (WISN) (http://www.who.int/hrh/resources/wisn_user_manual/en/, accessed 06 February 2017) can be useful for calculating the number of health workers and lay providers needed to provide adequate viral hepatitis testing services.

All personnel must be trained adequately, including those taking specimens, conducting testing, providing test reports, and data clerks and other auxiliary staff. All staff should have appropriate qualifications, such as certifications according to the national guidelines, and demonstrated proficiency in performing the tasks within their scope of work. **Both pre-service** and **in-service training**, including periodic refresher training, should be part of the training requirements for all testing services. In addition, regular **supportive supervision** and ongoing **mentoring** of all staff are essential.

15.6 Assuring the safety of testing services
15.6.1. Facilities and safety

It is critical that testing facilities are well designed and maintained. The testing site, including where counselling takes place, where specimens are taken and where the test is performed, should be clean and comfortable, with adequate lighting (for reading visually read assays) and free of any potential hazards. It is critical to guard against harm to any client, testing provider or other person at the testing site. This means that a **safe working environment** must be maintained by and for all staff, with necessary procedures in place. These procedures include universal precautions (assume that all specimens are potentially infectious), prevention of and/or response to needle-stick injuries or other occupational exposures, chemical and biological safety, spill containment, waste disposal and use of personal protective equipment.

It is imperative to follow the assay manufacturer's recommendations for the control of room temperature of areas where testing is performed. Where possible, testing should take place in climate-controlled areas. There must be proper **waste disposal** for biological (infectious and non-infectious), chemical and paper waste, and sharps.

15.7. Other practical considerations for testing
15.7.1. Testing at different levels of the health-care system

Testing for serological markers of HBV and HCV infection may take place at any level of the health-care system and for virological tests at levels 2 to 4. Fig. 15.2 depicts how testing services are typically organized, with the different assays formats that could feasibly be available at each of the levels when their operational characteristics and other factors such as need for phlebotomy are considered. The degree of physical infrastructure required for each assay format, such as the need for reliable electricity to store reagents and climate-controlled testing rooms to run tests, as well as the staff skills and competencies required, will determine how complex the assay can be for a given testing setting. With further expanded use of RDTs, more people could access testing at the primary care level (level 1).

FIG. 15.2. A tiered testing service, with test format menu and staff qualifications

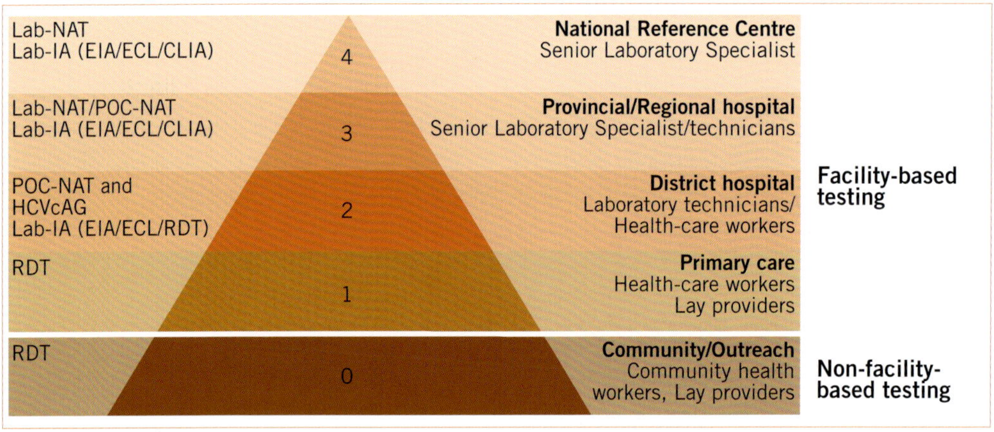

Level	Test formats	Setting / Staff	
4	Lab-NAT Lab-IA (EIA/ECL/CLIA)	**National Reference Centre** Senior Laboratory Specialist	Facility-based testing
3	Lab-NAT/POC-NAT Lab-IA (EIA/ECL/CLIA)	**Provincial/Regional hospital** Senior Laboratory Specialist/technicians	
2	POC-NAT and HCVcAG Lab-IA (EIA/ECL/RDT)	**District hospital** Laboratory technicians/ Health-care workers	
1	RDT	**Primary care** Health-care workers Lay providers	
0	RDT	**Community/Outreach** Community health workers, Lay providers	Non-facility-based testing

CLIA: chemiluminescence immunoassay; ECL: electrochemiluminescence immunoassay; EIA: enzyme immunoassay; RDT: rapid diagnostic test; Lab-NAT: laboratory-based nucleic acid testing; POC-NAT: nucleic acid testing at point of care

Source: Consolidated guidelines on HIV testing services. Geneva: WHO; 2015 *(11)*.

15.7.2. Specimen types and collection methods

Specimen integrity is critical to the accuracy of testing. Table 15.3 provides a broad summary of specimen types and processing requirements, but each manufacturer specifies in the instructions for use the recommended specimen collection procedures, the storage requirements and specimen stability after collection, and these instructions should always take precedence. Where the instructions for use do not include a certain specimen type within the intended use, it indicates that the assay manufacturer has not yet validated that specimen type for use with their assay.

Serum/plasma specimens are most commonly used for testing of HBV and HCV, both serological testing and NAT. However, taking whole blood specimens using **venepuncture requires technical skill and proficiency**, with the need for additional processing steps to generate serum/plasma from the venous whole blood, which requires a centrifuge and refrigerated storage facilities. Collection of **oral fluid** and **capillary whole blood** is less invasive than venepuncture. However, oral fluid testing is currently limited to serological tests, and may have lower sensitivity than testing performed on capillary whole blood or serum/plasma specimens.

TABLE 15.3. Specimen types and processing requirements

Specimen type	Time to processing/storage/time to testing
Venous whole blood Fresh whole blood collected by venepuncture	• Use the specimen immediately.
Serum Freshly collected whole blood is allowed to coagulate, and serum fraction is collected away from the clotted red blood cells.	• Collect whole blood, mix by hand 4–5 times immediately and let stand for the clot to form. • Process within 30 minutes of collection. • Store at 2–8 °C. Test within 5 days or as specified by the instructions for the assay to be used.
Plasma Freshly collected whole blood is added to recommended anticoagulant, such as EDTA, heparin or citrate. After centrifugation, plasma is separated.	• Collect whole blood, mix by hand 8–10 times immediately and centrifuge for up to 10 minutes. • Process within 6 hours of collection. • Store at 2–8 °C. Test within 5 days or as specified by the instructions for the assay to be used.
Capillary whole blood Capillary (finger-stick) whole blood is collected using a lancet and a specimen transfer device.	• Use the specimen immediately, with the specimen transfer device recommended by the instructions for use. • Note that the specimen transfer device may or may not include an anticoagulant. An anticoagulant contributes to accuracy.
Oral fluid Oral mucosal transudate (not saliva) is collected from the gums using a collection device.	• Use the specimen immediately, with the specimen transfer device recommended in the instructions for use.
Dried blood spot (DBS) Venous or capillary whole blood is applied to a filter paper by hanging drop or microcapillary action. Whole blood is later eluted from the filter paper and used for the test procedure.	• Store at 4 °C for up to 3 months, or at −20 °C for longer. • Use of specific assays with DBS should be validated by the manufacturer. If the manufacturer has not validated their assay for DBS, the use of DBS is considered "off-label", or unauthorized for returning medical results.

16. PRE-TEST AND POST-TEST COUNSELLING

This chapter discusses essential counselling and services prior to HBV and HCV testing. It also discusses post-test counselling for individuals who are diagnosed with chronic HBV or HCV infection, as well as those who test negative or who have an inconclusive result.

> ## Key points
>
> - The 5 "Cs" are essential for all hepatitis testing services: **consent, confidentiality, counselling, correct test results and connection** to hepatitis prevention, treatment and care.
>
> - Verbal consent is usually adequate, but all individuals should have an opportunity to refuse testing. Mandatory testing is never warranted.
>
> - Viral hepatitis testing services must ensure that all test results and client information are confidential. Although disclosure to supportive family members and health workers is often beneficial, this must be done only with the consent of the person being tested.
>
> - Everyone who is diagnosed positive for hepatitis B or hepatitis C should receive post-test counselling. People who test negative for hepatitis B or C will usually need only brief health information about how to prevent acquisition of viral hepatitis in the future, where and how to link to prevention services, as appropriate, and be offered HBV vaccination. People with significant ongoing risk such as PWID may need more active support and linkage to harm reduction services.
>
> - Connection or linkage to prevention, treatment and care is an essential component of viral hepatitis testing. Chapter 14 provides recommendations on approaches to improving linkages.

16.1. Promoting testing awareness

Depending on the current levels of knowledge and awareness of hepatitis in different countries and settings, general promotion and awareness campaigns for viral hepatitis testing and where it is available may be necessary. This may include promotion through the mass media, including radio, television, billboards and posters, the Internet and electronic social media. In other countries, promotional activities may need to focus on specific populations in whom viral hepatitis testing rates remain suboptimal, such as PWID. There is also a need for clear signs, printed information, posters that direct clients to where testing is available in health facilities (such as ANC, STI and TB clinics), the community or through mobile services and social media.

16.2. Creating an enabling environment

Critical enablers are strategies, activities and approaches (generally outside the purview of the health sector) that are key to the success of health sector interventions. Addressing such critical enablers as **reducing stigma and discrimination, empowering the community and reviewing certain national laws, policies and practice** can help strengthen interventions to support the uptake of viral hepatitis testing and linkages to prevention, care and treatment. In particular, it can improve the accessibility, acceptability, uptake, equitable coverage, quality, effectiveness and efficiency of viral hepatitis interventions, especially among populations that are reluctant to use or have limited access to current hepatitis testing, such as PWID.

16.3. The WHO 5 "Cs"

The WHO 5 "Cs" are principles that apply to all models of HIV and hepatitis testing and in all settings (Box 16.1) *(11)*.

Box 16.1 "The 5 Cs" for hepatitis testing services *(11)*

• **Consent.** People being tested for hepatitis B or C must give informed consent to be tested and counselled. Verbal consent is sufficient, and they should be informed of the process for testing and of their right to decline. Provision of information about testing and the need for consent can be delivered in a group setting, such as group health education, but clients should give consent in an individual and private manner. Health workers should carefully explain how a client can decline testing and ensure that no one coerces clients into being tested, and each person has a private opportunity to opt out of testing.

• **Confidentiality – ensuring a confidential setting and preserving confidentiality.** Testing must be confidential, meaning that what the provider and the client discuss will not be disclosed to anyone else without the expressed consent of the person being tested. Confidentiality applies not only to the test results and report of hepatitis status but also to any personal information, such as information concerning sexual behaviour and the use of illegal drugs. Hepatitis testing services should avoid practices that can inadvertently reveal a client's test results to others in the waiting room or in the health facility. Experiences with HIV testing services have shown that a lack of confidentiality discourages people from using testing services. Health workers and others who will provide testing may need special training and sensitization regarding the confidentiality of medical records.

Although confidentiality should always be respected, it should not be allowed to reinforce secrecy, stigma or shame. Counsellors should discuss, among other issues, whom the person may wish to inform and how they would like this to be done. Shared confidentiality with a partner or family members and health-care providers is often highly beneficial.

• **Counselling.** Pre-test information can be provided in a group setting, but all people should have the opportunity to ask questions in a private setting if they request it. All hepatitis testing must be accompanied by appropriate post-test counselling, based on the specific hepatitis test result and hepatitis status reported. QA mechanisms as well as supportive supervision and mentoring systems should be in place to ensure the provision of high-quality counselling.

• **Correct.** Providers of hepatitis testing should strive to provide high-quality testing services, and QA mechanisms should ensure that people receive a correct diagnosis. QA may include both internal and external measures, including support from the national reference laboratory. All people who receive a positive serological diagnosis of HBV or HCV should have a NAT to confirm the presence of viraemic infection and assess their need for care and treatment before starting antiviral therapy (Chapter 15).

• **Connection.** Linkage to prevention, treatment and care services should include effective and appropriate follow up, including long-term prevention and treatment support. Providing viral hepatitis testing where there is no access to care, or poor linkage to care and treatment, has limited benefit for those with hepatitis (Chapter 14).

16.4. Providing pre-test information

With the increasing availability of RDTs, many people will receive their initial serology test results on the same day as testing. Therefore, intensive pre-test counselling is not needed and may create barriers to service delivery. Depending on local conditions and resources, programmes may provide pre-test information through individual or group information sessions and through media such as posters, brochures, websites and short video clips shown in waiting rooms. When testing children and adolescents, information should be presented in an age-appropriate way to ensure comprehension.

Offering or recommending viral hepatitis testing to a client or a group of clients includes providing clear and concise information on:

- *viral hepatitis and the benefits of testing* for hepatitis B or C; and the meaning of a positive and negative test result;

- *a brief description of prevention options*;

- *the confidentiality of the test result,* as well as any information shared by the client;

- *the potential negative consequences of testing* to the client in settings where certain sexual or injecting drug use behaviour is stigmatized or even criminalized, or where a positive test could result in discrimination, for example, with regard to employment or with insurance policies where there may be financial consequences of either taking a test or of a positive result. In addition, the practical implications of a positive test result should be explained, including when there is no treatment currently available.

16.5. Post-test counselling and services

16.5.1. For those who test positive

Health workers, professional counsellors, social workers and trained lay providers can provide counselling. The information and counselling that health workers or others should provide to HBV- or HCV-positive clients is listed below. However, counselling should always be responsive to and tailored to the unique situation of each individual.

- *Explain the test results and diagnosis.*

- *Provide clear information on further tests* required to confirm viraemic infection and stage of liver disease, indications for treatment for both HBV and HCV and its benefits, as well as where and how to obtain the appropriate care and treatment (and advice if treatment is not currently available).

- *Make an active referral for viral hepatitis clinical care* for a specific time and date, i.e. tester makes an appointment or if services are co-located, accompanies the client to an appointment.

- *Provide information on how to prevent transmission of infection.* Preventive measures include HBV vaccination of non-immune clients, family members (including children), and sexual partners.

- *Counselling on lifestyle.* This includes assessment of alcohol consumption and advice on alcohol reduction (the WHO ASSIST package includes Alcohol, Smoking and Substance Involvement Screening Test)*(410)*, diet and physical activity.

- *Discuss possible disclosure of the result* and the risks and benefits of disclosure, particularly among couples and partners. Offer couples counselling to support mutual disclosure.

- *Encourage and offer HBV and HCV testing for family members,* including children, and sexual partners. This can be done individually, through couples testing or partner notification.

- *Provide additional referrals for prevention, counselling, support* and other services, as appropriate. These could include, for example, HIV, TB, STI diagnosis and treatment, contraception, antenatal care, reducing alcohol use, OST, access to sterile needles and syringes, and brief safe sex counselling.

- *Considerations in special populations.* In certain populations, such as PWID or those with mental health problems, intensified post-test counselling combined with follow-up counselling by referral to community health workers and to other services such as OST should be included in post-test counselling. A peer counsellor may particularly help people understand the diagnosis and support linkage to care and treatment by serving as a "peer navigator", who assists with finding, choosing and obtaining a full range of services, and can potentially increase the proportion of people who start treatment. Chapter 18 addresses considerations for testing in specific populations, e.g. pregnant and postpartum women, adolescents, and children.

16.5.2. For those who test negative

Individuals who test negative for HBV or HCV infection should receive brief health information about their test results. In general, a lengthy counselling session is not necessary and may divert counselling resources that are needed by those who test positive. Counselling for those who test negative should include the following, particularly in high-prevalence settings:

- *an explanation of the negative test result;*

- *an offer of HBV vaccination* and education on methods to prevent acquisition, and referral to harm reduction prevention services, as appropriate;

- *repeat testing for HCV* based on the client's level of recent exposure and/or ongoing risk of exposure. The majority of individuals do not require retesting to verify a negative test, particularly in the absence of any ongoing risk. However, certain individuals who test negative warrant retesting because of an ongoing risk, especially for HCV, but also for HBV if they have not yet been vaccinated. These include the following: persons from high-risk populations, such as PWID, sex workers and MSM; persons with a known HBsAg- or HCV RNA-positive partner or family member; pregnant women in high-prevalence settings (at each pregnancy); individuals seen for a diagnosis or treatment of HIV or STIs;

- *encouraging the client to return for a further test* to confirm the diagnosis when the hepatitis status is inconclusive

17. SERVICE DELIVERY APPROACHES FOR VIRAL HEPATITIS TESTING – examples from the field

This chapter summarizes the different facility- and community-based testing approaches available, i.e. where to test, and supports implementation of the recommendations on who to test for viral hepatitis in Chapters 6 and 7, with examples of their use in the field in different populations and settings. Chapter 19 provides a strategic framework to guide countries' decision-making on selecting testing approaches.

Key points

- Viral hepatitis testing can be delivered in different populations and different settings through both health-care facility-based testing and community-based testing.

- Many of these approaches have successfully increased the coverage and impact of HIV testing, and can be applied to the delivery of viral hepatitis testing.

- **Health-care facilities for testing** are primary care clinics and outpatient clinics that include specialist clinics such as HIV, STI and TB clinics, antenatal clinics, OST services, as well as inpatient wards in district, provincial and regional hospitals, and private clinical services. **Community-based testing** can be offered through outreach/mobile, home-based or door-to-door approaches, in schools and other educational establishments, and in workplaces, places of worship, parks, bars and other venues.

- Effective health system programme practices that may be appropriate for increasing access to hepatitis testing in some settings include **integration with other health services** (e.g. HIV), **decentralization of testing** to primary care facilities and outside the health system (e.g. workplaces, schools, places of worship), and **task-sharing of testing responsibilities** to other health workers, including trained lay providers.

- Countries need to identify the most strategic mix of facility- and community-based testing opportunities (as well as the use of integration, decentralization and task-sharing) to best reach those with undiagnosed infection and populations at high risk (*see* Chapter 19).

17.1. Health-care facility-based testing and provider-initiated testing and counselling

Health facility-based viral hepatitis testing refers to testing provided in a health facility or laboratory setting. There are several approaches to facility-based testing.

Provider or practitioner-initiated testing and counselling (PITC) denotes testing that is routinely offered at a health facility *(411)*, as well as for persons who request testing or who exhibit clinical signs, symptoms or laboratory results that could indicate HBV or HCV infection. It includes provision of pre-test information and obtaining consent, with the option for individuals to decline testing. Although voluntary counselling and testing (VCT) in stand-alone facilities was an early model for delivering HIV testing, it was recognized that offering testing in clinical sites as part of general medical care through PITC *(411)* resulted in increased HIV testing uptake, coverage and case detection. It also helped normalize testing by removing the potential reluctance of clients to request a test *(11, 411)*. PITC for hepatitis can be implemented and integrated in a number of clinical settings, as summarized below, and these represent major opportunities for scaling up viral hepatitis testing.

HIV clinics. In many populations and high-risk groups, prevalence of HIV and HBV or HCV is high, and there are also high rates of HIV/HBV or HIV/HCV coinfection *(88)*. Existing HIV and ART programmes provide an important opportunity to integrate testing for viral hepatitis with that for HIV (*see* Box 17.1).

Box 17.1. Integrated HIV/hepatitis testing

Médecins Sans Frontières (MSF) India. The MSF team in collaboration with the National AIDS Control Organization in India provided integrated HIV/TB/HCV services. Counsellors experienced in HIV testing and adherence counselling have also been trained to provide HCV pre-test counselling, HCV viral load testing, genotyping and FibroScan® for staging of liver fibrosis. Of the 1367 HIV-infected persons who were tested, 383 (28%) were HCV antibody seropositive.

Source: Hepatitis Testing Innovation Contest, 2016

TB clinics. Some populations who are at high risk for HBV and HCV infection are often also at risk for TB, e.g. PWID, prisoners, migrants and persons coinfected with HIV. WHO already recommends routine HIV testing for all TB patients (both active and presumptive cases) *(412)*, and this has proven highly acceptable *(413)*. Integrating HBV and HCV testing as part of a comprehensive package of care for TB patients should be both feasible and acceptable, particularly in settings and populations where the prevalence of TB and viral hepatitis is high.

STI clinics. HBV and HIV, and to a lesser extent HCV, are all sexually transmissible infections, and services providing care for STIs are therefore a key entry point for both HIV and viral hepatitis prevention and treatment services. New acquisition of STIs, such as gonorrhoea and syphilis, indicate recent unprotected sex and can help identify people at a heightened risk of acquisition of HIV and viral hepatitis. WHO already recommends routinely offering HIV testing for persons diagnosed with other STIs *(414)*, with a high uptake of testing *(415, 416)*. Extension to include targeted HBV and HCV testing is also likely to be feasible and acceptable.

Drug treatment and harm reduction services. Many innovative models of care to provide integrated hepatitis and OST services for PWID in community drug treatment services have been developed and effectively implemented, mostly in developed countries *(196, 362, 377, 417–419)*. Many of these programmes provide additional interventions, including education, harm reduction, mental health services, other general medical services, and direct provision of referrals to care and treatment. These models can provide a framework for lower-income countries to expand viral hepatitis testing and treatment for at-risk populations.

Inpatient and outpatient hospital settings present a further opportunity for testing in patients with symptoms or laboratory test findings, such as unexplained abnormal liver function tests that may be indicative of viral hepatitis infection. Testing in hospitals, particularly in low- or concentrated-epidemic settings, has proven effective in HIV case-finding in Europe *(420)*. Testing in hospital emergency departments has also been recently piloted in Europe and the United States (*see* Box 17.2) *(421)*.

Box 17.2. Using emergency departments to promote testing

The **Barts Health NHS Trust, London,** United Kingdom, "Going Viral" campaign brought together health authorities, pharmaceutical companies, and national media to promote a testing initiative for bloodborne viruses (HIV/HBV/HCV) in nine emergency departments. In addition to promotion in the emergency department, social media celebrity endorsements and television coverage were used. Of 7800 individuals having blood drawn in the emergency department, 2118 (27%) agreed to be tested, and 39 individuals with HCV and 15 with HBV were identified. Approximately half were previously unaware of their diagnosis, and 41 (76%) of these were linked to care, and attended at least one follow-up clinic. (http://bartshealth.nhs.uk/).

Source: Hepatitis Testing Innovation Contest, 2016

Primary-care settings may be more accessible and less stigmatizing than hospital-based clinics, particularly for high-risk and vulnerable populations such as PWID. Targeted case-finding of people with a history of injecting drug use can increase the number of people who are offered and accept HCV testing *(422)*. Studies also show that multidisciplinary care with integration of other services (e.g. drug and alcohol support, psychiatric services) at the same primary-care setting are acceptable and particularly effective for these populations, who often have multiple health comorbidities and complex needs *(417, 423–425)*. Peer-led models, or provider-led models with peer support, can be particularly effective in enabling integration of services in one place in a way that is acceptable to certain high-risk groups such as PWID. Electronic medical records (EMR) have been successfully used to identify and flag higher-risk patients for viral hepatitis testing in several primary-care clinic and hospital-based programmes (*see* Box 17.3).

> **Box 17.3. Use of electronic medical records (EMRs) to flag higher-risk primary care patients for testing**
>
> **National Nurse Care Consortium, Philadelphia, United States.** Five Philadelphia primary health centres have integrated HCV testing and linkage to care within community primary-care services. The EMRs were used to identify testing eligibility and expedite laboratory requisitions. A total of 9225 HCV tests were performed between October 2012 and January 2016. Of these, 1114 (12.1%) were HCV antibody positive and 1057 (95%) also had HCV RNA testing, of whom 765 (72%) were positive. Of these 765, 512 (67%) had a follow-up HCV medical evaluation and 110 (22%) received treatment. (www.nncc.us)
>
> *Source:* Hepatitis Testing Innovation Contest, 2016

Paediatric and adolescent clinics may be important settings for identifying cases of previously undiagnosed hepatitis B or C infections, particularly in high-prevalence countries. Offering testing to all children whose mother or father has either HBV or HCV infection, and to those with symptoms or laboratory findings that could be indicative of viral hepatitis infection may identify many infections. This could be integrated in clinics where PITC for HIV is already provided.

Routine testing in antenatal clinics (ANC) is a key opportunity to reduce the global burden of HBV disease, which is primarily propagated through ongoing MTCT in high-prevalence resource-limited settings. Testing for HBsAg enables women to have knowledge of their HBV serostatus for their own health, and for their offspring to benefit from interventions to prevent MTCT, including birth dose and infant HBV vaccination, use of hepatitis B immune globulin (HBIG), and antiviral therapy. PITC for HBV offered routinely in ANC has proven feasible and acceptable in several settings. However, although many countries recommend routine screening, the proportion actually screened in many high-burden LMICs remains low *(157)*. The additional cost of also testing pregnant women for HCV alongside HIV and HBV is likely to be low (*see* Box 17.4).

> **Box 17.4. Antenatal clinic testing for hepatitis B infection**
>
> Antenatal testing is a key opportunity to prevent MTCT with neonatal vaccination and use of HBIG and antiviral therapy.
>
> **Yunnan AIDS Initiative in China.** This nongovernmental organization implemented a combined HIV, HBV and syphilis testing campaign in ANC, labour and delivery units throughout the province. An opt-out testing model for the women was used and partners were also offered testing. The Chinese government has recently adopted routine HIV, HBV and syphilis testing in ANC in over 1000 counties nationwide after the success of the Yunnan AIDS Initiative and several other demonstration projects.
>
> *Source:* Hepatitis Testing Innovation Contest, 2016

17.2. Community-based testing

Community-based testing can complement facility-based approaches, which may fail to reach certain high-risk populations, especially PWID, who are often marginalized because of stigma and discrimination or legal sanctions, as well as those in remote or rural areas, including pregnant women with limited access to facility-based testing. There is some evidence that offering hepatitis testing in community settings may increase testing acceptance and uptake, achieve earlier diagnosis, reach first-time testers and people who seldom use clinical services *(194, 422)*. However, the same barriers encountered in ensuring linkage to HIV prevention, care and treatment services will need to be addressed. Such outreach methods aimed at HIV prevention have been shown to be particularly effective in engaging with hard-to-reach PWID populations, and decreasing injection and sexual risk behaviours *(426)* (*see* Box 17.5).

Mobile/Outreach testing approaches include outreach to community sites through mobile vans or tents, at community sites such as churches, mosques or other faith settings, in places of entertainment such as bars and clubs, at cruising sites. Such services may be offered on a regular schedule, at night ("moonlight testing"), or as a one-time or occasional promoted event, linked to public events, such as sports events, music performances, theatre, agricultural fairs and holiday festivals.

Door-to-door/home-based testing takes place in the home. There are two main models: (i) testing that is offered door to door and provided to all consenting individuals, couples or families in a geographical area; and (ii) testing that is offered to households with an index patient (i.e. persons known to have HIV, viral hepatitis or active or presumptive TB), with consent obtained from the index patient before the home visit. Door-to-door testing during the daytime may reach only people who are not working and younger children, while services during the evening or on weekends may increase uptake among others, such as men.

> **Box 17.5 Reaching people who inject drugs**
>
> Tailored HCV testing and linkage to care services for PWID are a critical part of delivering HCV services. Integration of HCV testing into PWID services (including drug dependence treatment services, needle and syringe services, PWID community health services) is effective in a range of settings.
>
> **Care & Cure Service Center (CCSC) Kerinchi in Kuala Lumpur, Malaysia**. A methadone clinic screened and counselled individuals for HCV. Their programme collaborated with public hospitals, facilitating service integration after testing. Of 544 methadone clinic attendees 304 (55%) have been evaluated and tested for HCV antibody. Of those, 235 (77%) tested positive and 81 (34.5%) were referred for clinical care. (www.ceria.um.edu.my/)
>
> **Testing camps: Community Network for Empowerment (CONE) in Manipur, India.** As part of a province-wide campaign to identify more cases of viral hepatitis, a community organization partnered with provincial government and pharmaceutical companies to establish testing camps. They provided free screening and HCV RNA confirmatory tests together with liver scans for staging of liver fibrosis. Of 1011 individuals (including PWID, people living with HIV, and general clinic attendees) tested for HCV, 463 were confirmed to be HCV RNA positive. Linkage to treatment is now under way since DAAs have become available. (www.conemanipur.net)
>
> *Source:* Hepatitis Testing Innovation Contest, 2016

National testing campaigns are nationwide efforts to increase access to and uptake of testing. Some have focused on testing in facilities while others have used a community-based approach or a combination of the two. Outcomes have varied with regard to coverage of different population groups, linkage and cost–effectiveness. A national or regional hepatitis testing campaign has the potential to reach a significant proportion of the population, which includes both those known to be at risk as well as those not at risk for HBV or HCV infection (*see* Box 17.6). However, experience with national HIV campaigns has shown that they can be expensive, and that a substantial number of people with HIV remain undiagnosed. In addition, linkage to care and treatment from campaigns has been problematic.

> **Box 17.6 Reaching general populations through community-based and primary clinic testing**
>
> **Egyptian Liver Research Institute, Mansoura, Egypt.** In El Othmanya village in northern Egypt, a social marketing and community mobilization campaign was implemented to promote household testing for hepatitis B and C among all adolescents and adults. The majority (98%, 3500/3573) of household members were tested and 270 (7.7%) were confirmed HCV RNA positive and 8 (0.22%) HBV DNA positive. Treatment-eligible cases were linked to care at the Egyptian Liver Hospital and treatment costs were covered through community fund-raising or the government health insurance system. The model is being scaled up in 30 other villages. (http://www.nrc.sci.eg/)
>
> **Ishikawa Prefecture and Kanazawa University Hospital, Japan.** Since 2001, the government has provided free hepatitis testing at five-year intervals for all citizens aged between 40 and 70 years. A total of 240 180 individuals, or 38% of the target population in Ishikawa prefecture, were tested. The programme also provides at least annual follow up of all diagnosed patients for liver fibrosis staging and treatment. (http://www.m-kanazawa.jp/english/index.html)
>
> **Prevention of Liver Fibrosis and Cancer in Africa (PROLIFICA), Gambia.** Is the first community- and facility-based screen and treat programme for HBV infection in sub-Saharan Africa and offers testing to all rural and urban inhabitants aged 30 years or older in the western part of Gambia. HBsAg screening was accepted by 68.9% of 8170 adults and 81.4% of 6832 blood donors, and was positive in 495 (8.8%) of individuals in the community and 721 (13%) of blood donors. All individuals who tested HBsAg positive were referred for comprehensive outpatient assessment to determine eligibility for treatment. Linkage to care was high in the community (81.3%) but lower (41.6%) among blood donors, and treatment eligibility was 4.4% and 9.7%, respectively. (https://www.prolifica.org.uk/)
>
> *Source:* Hepatitis Testing Innovation Contest, 2016

Mass media and social media. Knowledge of hepatitis testing and availability is limited in many countries, and there is a need for promotion and awareness campaigns in the general population. Some countries and programmes promote viral hepatitis testing and education through the mass media, including radio, television, billboards and posters, the Internet and electronic social media (*see* Box 17.7). This approach has also been used to facilitate more targeted and efficient screening in regions of low prevalence. This also applies to testing in health facilities, in the community and through mobile services (*see* Box 17.7).

> **Box 17.7 Use of Internet and social media to promote testing in the general population**
>
> **Public Health Service of Amsterdam, Netherlands.** The campaign goal was to motivate at-risk groups to independently assess their HCV risk, using an online risk assessment tool developed by the Amsterdam Public Health Service. Participants received a laboratory form for anonymous HCV testing via the website if the tool rated them as being at high risk. Approximately 9700 individuals took the online risk assessment, 1500 were offered testing, and 28% of these used the organization's testing facility. The HCV antibody positivity rate was 3.6%. Test results were also available online along with invitations for confirmatory testing. (www.ggd.amsterdam.nl)
>
> *Source:* Hepatitis Testing Innovation Contest, 2016

Workplace testing provides employed men and women access to testing, who otherwise might have limited access to clinical services because they need to take time off work to seek health care. Concerns with workplace testing include the potential for coercion, breaches in confidentiality, and weak linkages to services, and care must be taken that this approach is not promoted where it is likely to be abused. For example, 60% of HIV testing in the Middle East and North Africa region is undertaken through workplace testing and work visa procedures, and is generally mandatory *(427)*. It should not therefore be considered an effective model for scale up of hepatitis testing. However, workplace testing for HIV and TB with onward linkage to HIV and TB services has been successfully implemented in several high-burden settings *(428–430)*. Many workplace health programmes do not include hepatitis programmes, creating an opportunity for expanding workplace testing (*see* Box 17.8).

> **Box 17.8 Workplace testing**
>
> **Asian Liver Center, Stanford University, United States.** This project partnered with 42 corporations to increase awareness of HBV and HCV testing in several countries. An online tool (www.hepbhra.org) was developed, which allowed individuals in the workplace to assess their risk of hepatitis B infection and make decisions about being tested. (http://liver.stanford.edu/).
>
> *Source:* Hepatitis Testing Innovation Contest, 2016

Testing in schools, colleges or other educational establishments can facilitate access to testing among sexually active young persons by bringing services to students who may find it challenging to seek HIV or hepatitis testing during school hours, and be otherwise hard to reach, as they do not use health services or community services. The service may also provide sexual health education and counselling on risk reduction. In South Africa, a national campaign provides HIV testing to students aged 12 years and older in schools *(431)*. However, school-based HIV testing remains controversial, and few countries have established such programmes. Further evaluation is needed to understand issues of confidentiality, linkage to care and adolescents' experiences with and expectations of school-based testing for both viral hepatitis and HIV, as well as the impact and acceptability of testing among university students.

Testing in prisons and other correctional system settings is a potentially effective way to expand testing uptake among high-risk populations, as many prisoners are at increased risk of acquiring hepatitis B and C infection. There are also additional ethical and regulatory procedures involved in establishing testing programmes in prison settings. Several effective case studies demonstrate how hepatitis testing can be undertaken in prison and justice system settings (*see* Box 17.9).

Box 17.9 Prison and correctional hepatitis testing

St Vincent's Hospital Melbourne and Department of Justice and Regulation, Victorian State Government, Australia. HCV prevalence among prisoners in Victoria state is high at 25% and new transmissions also occur within prisons. A state-wide programme was initiated with the goal of eliminating transmission of viral hepatitis within its thirteen prisons through the assessment, education and management of prisoners with chronic viral hepatitis. All prisoners are screened for viral hepatitis on prison entry or transfer. Prisoners who are seropositive are referred to the Victorian State-wide Prison Hepatitis Program for further assessment and initiation of antiviral therapy supervised by trained clinical nurse consultants during visits every 2–4 weeks. This programme is integrated into the prison primary care system and uses telemedicine for consultations with two part-time hepatologists, and provision of DAAs since March 2015. (http://www.svhm.org.au/)

Source: Hepatitis Testing Innovation Contest, 2016

17.3. Good practices for delivery of effective viral hepatitis testing services

17.3.1. Effective health system programming practices

Delivery models for viral hepatitis testing, care and treatment can be informed and strengthened by experience from the global scale up of HIV testing and treatment. The WHO-recommended effective health programming practices of ***integration*** with other health services; ***decentralization*** to primary health-care facilities as well as outside the health system (e.g. workplaces, schools, places of worship); and ***task-shifting*** of responsibilities to increase the role of trained lay providers were originally developed to improve the delivery of HIV testing *(11) (see Glossary)*. Inclusion of one or more of these practices may improve the accessibility of hepatitis testing, and onward linkage to services and support in some settings. With the availability of simplified viral hepatitis diagnostic tests and treatment regimens, decentralization and task-shifting or -sharing in particular can be increasingly used in service delivery models to scale up hepatitis testing and treatment, especially in settings where there is limited access to hospital facilities and laboratory services *(432)*.

17.3.2. Integration of viral hepatitis testing with other services

Integration involves not only providing related services in a single setting, but also linking recording and reporting systems to share information and referrals between settings and providers. There is already a range of clinical services for which WHO recommends the integration of HIV testing, and this may also apply to hepatitis testing in some settings (*see* Table 17.1). These include clinical services for TB, HIV, maternal and child health, sexual and reproductive health (STI clinics), mental health and harm reduction programmes for PWID, migrant and refugee services, and persons in prisons *(5, 6, 25, 28, 432)*. Integration with HIV testing and treatment services will be particularly appropriate in HBV and HCV epidemic settings where the HIV prevalence is also high.

Table 17.1. Potential populations and programmes for integration to promote hepatitis testing

Disease	High-risk groups and potential programme integration
Hepatitis B	• Infants of infected mothers (delivery units, maternal and child health [under-5 and immunization] clinics) • Children in endemic regions (maternal and child health [under-5 and immunization] clinics) • Sexual transmission in adults (STI and HIV clinics) • People who inject drugs (harm reduction and drug treatment services) • Health-care workers (occupational health)
Hepatitis C	• People who have received unsafe therapeutic injections/blood products (health promotion) • People who inject drugs (harm reduction and drug treatment services) • Men who have sex with men (STI and HIV clinics) • Health-care workers (occupational health)

Source: Adapted from: Mihigo R, Nshimirimana D, Hall A, Kew M, Wiersma S, Clements CJ. Control of viral hepatitis infection in Africa: are we dreaming? Vaccine. 2013;31 (2):341–6.

The primary purpose of such integration is to make HBV, HCV and HIV testing more convenient for people coming to health facilities for other reasons, and so expand the reach and uptake of viral hepatitis testing. For the patient, integration of hepatitis testing into other health services may facilitate addressing other health needs at the same time, saving time and money. For the health system, integration may reduce duplication of services and improve coordination, for example, in stock management, overall efficiency and cost–effectiveness.

The goal of programme collaboration is to create integrated delivery systems that best facilitate access to and increase the impact of hepatitis testing, treatment and other health services. Aspects of coordination across programmes that need consideration include: mobilizing, allocating and sharing resources (including multitasking and task-shifting of human resources to increase the availability of highly skilled workers); training, mentoring and supervising health workers; procuring and managing medicines, test kits and other medical supplies; maintaining the quality of testing; and reducing stigma and discrimination *(433)*.

17.3.3. Decentralization of hepatitis testing services

Decentralization of services refers to delivery of services provided in peripheral health facilities, community-based venues and locations beyond urban hospital sites, nearer to patients' homes. This may reduce transportation costs and waiting times experienced in central hospitals and, therefore, improve uptake of testing. Decentralization of HIV treatment services, in high-burden LMICs was a key component of the global scale up of HIV services and successfully improved uptake of testing and reduced loss to follow up *(402)*. To date, delivery of viral hepatitis testing and treatment has in general relied on specialist-led centralized models of care in hospital settings *(432)*. Currently, there are only a few successful models of decentralized viral hepatitis testing and treatment for hard-to-reach populations and general populations at high risk (*see* Box 17.10). With the development of simpler diagnostic tests for HBV and HCV, and simpler and more effective treatment regimens for HCV, decentralization has the potential to also increase the uptake of hepatitis testing.

> **Box 17.10 Decentralization**
>
> **In Taiwan**, a community-based outreach model delivering free testing for HBV and HCV and targeting the general population has been successfully implemented since 1996, and identified a high overall seroprevalence of both HBV and HCV (17.3% and 4.4%, respectively) and significant geographical variations in prevalence *(434)*.
>
> *Source:* Hepatitis Testing Innovation Contest, 2016

Decentralization of services, however, may not always be appropriate for or acceptable to potential users. In some settings, centralized viral hepatitis services can provide greater anonymity than neighbourhood services for high-risk populations or others who fear stigma and discrimination. Also, in some low-prevalence settings, decentralizing hepatitis testing may be inefficient and costly. Context, needs, access to laboratory infrastructure and tests, and overall costs and benefits should inform decisions about where hepatitis testing should be decentralized. Decentralization of testing services will also require access to quality-assured RDTs, and DBS specimen collection and analysis.

17.3.4. Task-shifting or -sharing in delivery of hepatitis testing

Many countries, including those affected by HBV, HCV and HIV epidemics, continue to face shortages of trained health workers. Task-shifting is a pragmatic response to health workforce shortages. It seeks to increase the effectiveness and efficiency of available personnel and so enable the existing workforce to provide testing services to more people.

Several systematic reviews from different areas of health care support the general conclusion that good health outcomes can be achieved by devolving tasks to nurses and lay or community health workers *(435–438)*, with appropriate training and supervision. Task-shifting has been adopted for over a decade to expand HIV testing across the Americas *(441)*, Europe *(442, 443)*, sub-Saharan Africa *(444–449)* and Asia *(450)*, especially in resource-limited settings where there is a shortage of health-care professionals *(438)*. WHO now recommends that lay providers who are trained and supervised can independently perform HIV counselling and testing using RDTs *(11, 439)*. HIV testing in pregnancy can also be promoted through prescription of ART by nurses *(440)*.

In a similar way, task-shifting may also be important for scale up of hepatitis testing, particularly in settings with high HBV or HCV prevalence in the general population or subpopulations (*see* Box 17.11). Incorporation of viral hepatitis testing into existing task-shifting models of care providing HIV services could be an effective and cost–effective means of fulfilling these objectives. Peer-led interventions have also been effective in increasing viral hepatitis testing, care and treatment for marginalized groups of PWID. In addition to providing services, peers can act as role models and offer non-judgemental and respectful support that may contribute to reducing stigma, facilitating access to services and improving their acceptability *(25)*. However, increasing task-shifting and broadening the scope of responsibilities of trained lay providers will not alone fully rectify staff shortages and poor-quality services.

Box 17.11 Task-shifting

There is emerging evidence from high-income countries that task-shifting can help deliver effective HCV-related services to vulnerable key populations with outcomes comparable to specialist-level care *(346, 451)*. **In British Columbia, Canada**, a nurse-coordinated but specialist-supported model of care with specific training and clear protocols resulted in good HCV treatment outcomes in rural and small urban centres *(452)*, and in prisons in **Australia** *(451)*. Nurses were responsible for patient assessments and education as well as making referrals to other appropriate services according to patients' needs. In the ECHO programme, **New Mexico, United States**, primary health-care providers successfully provided high-quality HCV treatment to patients in rural areas and prisons *(346)*.

Source: Hepatitis Testing Innovation Contest, 2016

17.4. Diagnostic innovations to promote access to testing

Advances in hepatitis virus detection technology have created new opportunities for enhancing hepatitis testing, as well as monitoring the response to treatment. Future directions and innovations in testing include simplified single virological assay testing algorithms, near patient or POC assays for NAT and core antigen, DBS sampling (Chapter 13), multiplex/polyvalent platforms, and self-testing.

Simplified testing algorithms. Simplifying testing algorithms will be critical to ensuring affordability and the success of scaling up testing. Potential future testing approaches for HCV infection are the adoption of a less expensive and more manageable single virological test for both diagnosis and confirmation of viraemia *(453)*. However, this may only ever be cost–effective in high-prevalence settings and high-risk populations.

Near patient or POC testing. The development of reliable, accurate, practical and affordable near patient tests will be crucial for expanding hepatitis testing services, especially in community-based settings. POC technologies for viral hepatitis include molecular NAT-based tests for diagnosis and treatment monitoring. These emerging POC devices are able to perform conventional laboratory molecular testing (qualitative and quantitative) in field settings; are easier to use than the laboratory-based NAT assays, as they require minimum training and hands-on time; can be operated on battery or conventional power source; do not require phlebotomy; and provide a result within 2 hours. They include cartridge-based HCV RNA assays, which can be used with existing diagnostic platforms developed for TB or HIV early infant diagnosis and viral load monitoring, but HCVcAg POC platforms are also in development. They offer the possibility of a same-day diagnosis of viraemic infection, either alone or when combined with an HCV antibody RDT, as well as test of cure.

Multiplex and multi-disease analysers. Multiplex or multi-disease analysers allow for integrated testing of hepatitis B and C alongside other pathogens, e.g. HIV and syphilis, and can leverage technology developed for other infectious disease programmes. Key advantages include the requirement for lower specimen volume, improved client flow with results for multiple pathogens available at the same time, and so fewer patient visits and transport costs. Multiplex RDTs are in development for anti-HIV/anti-HCV, anti-HIV/syphilis/anti-HCV, anti-HIV/syphilis/HBsAg and anti-HIV/anti-HCV/HBsAg. Data on their diagnostic accuracy and impact on patient-important outcomes are required before adoption.

Self-testing. Self-testing is a process in which an individual, who wants to know his or her status collects a specimen, performs a test and interprets the result themselves, often in private. HIV self-testing (HIVST) is now being conducted in many settings. Most studies report that HIVST is highly acceptable across a variety of populations *(454–456)*, and has increased uptake of testing among people not reached by other existing HIV testing services, many of whom are first-time testers *(21, 457)*. The experience with hepatitis self-testing is currently very limited, but it represents a potentially important approach to expand access to testing in the future.

18. TESTING ISSUES IN SPECIFIC POPULATIONS

This chapter addresses special considerations that apply to viral hepatitis testing in certain priority and high-risk or key populations. This includes PWID; persons in prisons or closed settings; MSM; sex workers; transgender people; persons living with HIV; TB-infected populations; migrant and mobile populations; health-care workers; couples, partners and household contacts; pregnant women; children; and adolescents.

18.1. Principles for testing in all populations

- Hepatitis testing must emphasize the WHO 5 "Cs". Mandatory, compulsory or coercive testing is never appropriate (*see* Chapter 16).

- All sites that provide hepatitis testing should have SOPs and ethical codes of conduct. They should protect client information and confidentiality, and should employ trained and supervised health workers (including lay providers).

- All HBV and HCV testing should follow WHO testing strategies and a validated national testing algorithm. Hepatitis testing should have appropriate QA and quality improvement (QI) mechanisms in place.

- Testing should be part of a care pathway that includes access to prevention, treatment and vaccination services. All persons who test positive for HBV and HCV should be linked to hepatitis care and treatment services.

- Priority for testing is to diagnose the undiagnosed as well as to identify those both in greatest need of treatment and at greatest risk of transmitting infection.

18.2. Principles for testing in key and high-risk populations

In some countries, HIV, HBV and HCV infections occur predominantly in certain key or high-risk populations, often via common routes of transmission. Key populations include PWID, MSM, people in prisons and other closed settings, sex workers and transgender people. These populations not only have an increased risk of infection, but their behaviours are often stigmatized, discriminated and criminalized. In almost all countries and settings, hepatitis testing for these key and priority populations is inadequate, and access to prevention, care and treatment services remains low.

- **Promotion of health equity and human rights** in hepatitis B and C testing is critical, as many of the affected populations such as PWID, prisoners, MSM, and sex workers are those who are systematically excluded from access to testing, treatment and care. Expanded testing and access should be fair, equitable and voluntary, and provided in a supportive environment free of stigma and discrimination.

- **Essential strategies to create an enabling environment** for access to hepatitis testing and treatment in these populations include: supportive legislation, policy and financial commitment, such as decriminalization of behaviours of key populations; addressing stigma and discrimination and violence against people from key populations; and community empowerment. In prisons, this can also include addressing additional systemic barriers contributing to transmission of viral hepatitis and other infectious diseases, such as confined unhygienic living spaces, lack of access to clean drinking water and adequate nutrition *(458)*.

- **Testing in prisons.** Prisons provide an opportunity to offer testing and treatment to marginalized populations that otherwise might have difficulties accessing care. However, there is a need to guard against the negative consequences of testing in prisons such as mandatory or coercive testing and segregation of prisoners. There are also often major challenges to continuity of care between prisons and the community. All people who test positive need to be linked to viral hepatitis care and treatment services on discharge.

- **Provision of a comprehensive package of prevention and treatment interventions.** The high prevalence of comorbidities (e.g. viral hepatitis/HIV coinfection, TB, mental health issues and polydrug use) in PWID and other high-risk populations means that the provision of comprehensive prevention, treatment, care and social services is important. WHO has outlined a comprehensive set of interventions and approaches for PWID *(140)*, prisoners *(459)*, MSM and sex workers *(27, 57)*. These include provision of condoms, STI screening, HBV vaccination, OST provision and needle–syringe programme (NSP), and referral for ART and antiviral therapy.

- **Full HBV vaccination** or adoption of a catch-up vaccination programme is recommended for certain populations at increased risk of HBV, including PWID, MSM *(26)*, sex workers and prisoners, without the need for prior HBsAg testing.

- **Provision of accessible testing and treatment services.**
  - **Integration of testing and service delivery.** To facilitate access, testing in certain populations such as PWID should be integrated, where possible, with delivery of other harm-reduction or drug dependency services and HIV testing *(460)*.

- **Training of health-care workers.** In many settings, health-care workers lack experience or training on how to provide inclusive and non-judgemental testing, and there are reports of discrimination against high-risk populations. Countries should prioritize the training of health workers so that they can provide acceptable services, better understand the needs of these populations, and be familiar with local support and prevention services. Similarly, services for transgender persons should be welcoming, with staff who are respectful and sensitive to transgender issues, and are knowledgeable about transgender medical concerns, such as the integration of hormone therapy and hepatitis care.

- **Testing and repeat testing.** Testing should be offered to not only current injecting drug users but to all persons who have ever injected drugs. Repeat screening is required in PWID and other groups such as MSM at ongoing risk of infection with a negative test. The possibility of reinfection after spontaneous clearance or successful treatment should also be considered. Those who have been previously infected should be retested using RNA testing, as the antibody remains positive after the first infection.

Further reading

* Consolidated guidelines on HIV prevention, diagnosis, treatment and care for key populations. Geneva: WHO; 2014 and update 2016 *(25)* describes essential services for key populations and interventions to reduce barriers to testing and linkage to care after testing. (http://www.who.int/hiv/pub/guidelines/keypopulations/en/)

* Integrating collaborative TB and HIV services within a comprehensive package of care for people who inject drugs. Geneva: WHO; 2016 *(461)*. (http://apps.who.int/iris/bitstream/10665/204484/1/9789241510226_eng.pdf?ua=1)

* Guidance on prevention of viral hepatitis B and C among people who inject drugs. Geneva: WHO 2012 (http://apps.who.int/iris/bitstream/10665/75357/1/9789241504041_eng.pdf) *(28)*

* WHO, UNODC, UNAIDS Technical guide for countries to set targets for universal access to HIV prevention, treatment and care for injecting drug users –2012 revision. Geneva: WHO 2013 (http://www.who.int/hiv/pub/idu/targets_universal_access/en/, accessed 08 July 2016) *(140)*.

*UNODC, ILO, UNDP, WHO, UNAIDS. HIV prevention, treatment and care in prisons and other closed settings: a comprehensive package of interventions. Vienna: UNODC; 2013 (http://www.who.int/hiv/pub/prisons/interventions_package/en/, accessed 08 July 2016) *(459)*.

*Prevention and treatment of HIV and other sexually transmitted infections for sex workers in low- and middle-income countries . Geneva: WHO; 2012. (https://www.unfpa.org/sites/default/files/pub-pdf/9789241504744_eng.pdf) *(27)*.

*Implementing comprehensive HIV/STI programmes with sex workers: practical approaches from collaborative interventions. Geneva: World Health Organization; 2013 (http://apps.who.int/iris/bitstream/10665/90000/1/9789241506182_eng.pdf) *(57)*.

18.3 Persons living with HIV

Concurrent infection with HIV usually results in more severe and progressive liver disease, and a higher incidence of cirrhosis, HCC and mortality *(462–465)*. HIV-infected persons are therefore a priority group for early diagnosis of viral hepatitis coinfection, and provision of both ART and specific antiviral therapy.

Implementation considerations

- **Comparable outcomes of DAA therapy have been seen in persons with HIV coinfection** as for those with HCV monoinfection, with cure rates higher than 95%, even for those with prior HCV treatment failure or advanced fibrosis *(5)*. Therefore, there is no longer a need to consider HIV/HCV-coinfected patients as a special, difficult-to-treat patient population.

- **HBV vaccination.** The risk of HBV infection may be higher in HIV-infected adults, and therefore all persons newly diagnosed with HIV should be screened for HBsAg and anti-HBs to identify those with CHB, and vaccinated if non-immune. Response to HBV vaccine may be lower in HIV-infected persons especially those with a low CD4 count. A schedule using four double (40 μg) doses of the vaccine provides a higher protective anti-HBs titre than the regular three 20 μg dose schedule *(466)*.

18.4 Tuberculosis-infected populations

Certain groups, such as PWID and people in prisons who at increased risk of HCV and HBV infection, are also at risk of infection with TB, largely because they live in regions and/or settings (e.g. prisons or regions of the world) that are endemic for these infections *(467, 468)*.

Implementation considerations

- **Supporting intensified tuberculosis case-finding at testing facilities.** Screening for active TB should be part of the clinical evaluation of patients being considered for HBV and/or HCV and HIV treatment. WHO recommends a four-symptom screening algorithm to rule out active TB *(412)*. In the absence of a cough, weight loss, fever and night sweats, active TB can be confidently ruled out. In the presence of these symptoms, further investigations for TB would be recommended.

- **Drug interactions.** Drug-induced liver injury is three- to sixfold higher in persons coinfected with HBV, HCV or HIV who are receiving antituberculosis drugs. All existing DAA combination regimens interact with rifampicin, but there are no serious interactions anticipated between sofosbuvir or daclatasvir and multidrug-resistant (MDR) or extensively drug-resistant (XDR)-TB regimens *(469)*.

18.5. Migrant and mobile populations

In some low-prevalence HBV and HCV regions, such as North America, Europe and Australia, the prevalence of viral hepatitis infection among persons born in high- and intermediate-endemic countries is higher, and reflects that in their country of origin. In other settings, minority ethnic groups and other mobile populations such as migrant workers, refugees, asylum seekers, fisher folk and lorry drivers, are particularly vulnerable to HBV, HCV and HIV infection. All these groups can be hard to reach and have difficulty in accessing health care for HIV or hepatitis testing services because of stigma, language differences, discrimination and legal barriers *(53)*. Displacement of populations through human trafficking may further complicate the provision of testing services *(53)*.

Implementation considerations

- Knowledge of the underlying prevalence of viral hepatitis as well as other important diseases of public health significance in migrants and refugees is key for an effective country programme.

- Barriers to testing uptake among migrant groups, such as language and cultural barriers, need to be addressed in order to increase uptake of testing *(193)*. There is evidence that provision of information and education on hepatitis B to migrant populations may improve knowledge about risk, screening and prevention *(470)*, but not necessarily lead to increased uptake of testing.

- Persons who have travelled to high-prevalence countries and had an invasive procedure, including tattoos, acupuncture, body piercings, with equipment that may not have been properly sterilized, or those who may have engaged in high-risk sexual behaviours or injecting drug use should also be considered for targeted testing.

18.6. Health-care workers

Due to the risks associated with occupational exposure to blood and body fluids, health-care workers are a population at risk for acquisition of both hepatitis B and C infection. Exposure to blood and bodily fluids can occur through needle-stick and other sharps injuries, contact with blood and bodily fluids through scratches, abrasions or burns on the skin as well as mucosal surfaces of the eyes, nose, or mouth through accidental splashes *(68)*. However, the largest proportion of occupational transmission of viral hepatitis is due to percutaneous injury via needles during vascular access *(66)*. The risk of HBV transmission with such exposure is estimated to be 6–30% and for HCV transmission around 1.8% *(68)*.

Implementation considerations

In all settings, testing for hepatitis B (and in many settings for hepatitis C) and the offer of HBV vaccination to health-care workers who are non-immune should be standard practice, but this is currently not widely implemented in LMICs.

- **Infection control and injection safety.** In settings where infection control practices and occupational health and safety standards are inadequate, testing initiatives should take place alongside improvements in safety standards and procedures to protect health-care workers against possible exposure.

- **Post-exposure prophylaxis.** In the event of exposure to HBV, post-exposure prophylaxis with HBV vaccine and HBIG should be made available for health-care workers exposed to HBV where the worker has not received vaccination or where the antibody response to HBV vaccination is unknown.

- **Early diagnosis and management** of chronic hepatitis B and C infection should be available to all health-care workers where occupational transmission of HBV or HCV has occurred. Those who are HBsAg positive and undertake exposure-prone procedures, such as surgeons, gynaecologists, nurses, phlebotomists, personal care attendants and dentists, should be considered for HBV antiviral therapy to reduce direct transmission to others, and DAA therapy for HCV.

18.7. Couples, partners, family members and household contacts

Testing of couples and partners, family members and household contacts of persons with CHB infection, may be an efficient and effective way of identifying additional people with HBV infection who can also benefit from treatment and monitoring. This may also enable adoption of prevention strategies by the couple or family members (e.g. HBV vaccination, condom use, safe injecting practices) *(471)*. Although the risk of HCV transmission to household contacts and sexual partners among heterosexual and HIV-negative MSM partners is low, there is a small but increased risk among sexual partners of PWID and MSM who engage in high-risk sexual behaviours or are HIV positive. An increasing number of countries offer couples and partner HIV testing *(471)* in various settings, including ANC, community-based TB services, and HIV/ART clinics, and this can also inform the service delivery of partner testing for viral hepatitis.

Implementation considerations

- **Couples counselling** requires additional training and enhanced counselling skills. Providers must be aware of the potential for intimate partner-based violence and should accept people's decisions not to test with their partners.

Testing for couples who ask to be tested together promotes mutual disclosure of status and increases adoption of prevention measures, especially in the case of discordant couples.

> **Further reading**
>
> Guidance on couples HIV testing and counselling – including antiretroviral therapy for treatment and prevention in serodiscordant couples: recommendations for a public health approach. Geneva: WHO; 2012 (http://apps.who.int/iris/bitstream/10665/44646/1/9789241501972_eng.pdf?ua=1) *(471).*

18.8. Pregnant women

Hepatitis B infection. Universal HBV testing in pregnant women already occurs in many parts of the world, but remains suboptimal in resource-limited settings *(157)*. Box 18.1 summarizes the existing WHO guidelines on HBV infection prevention in newborns *(6)*, but the most important preventive strategy is to deliver the first dose of hepatitis B vaccine as soon as possible after birth, preferably within 24 hours followed by at least two timely subsequent doses. Recent studies have suggested that there may also be a role for antiviral therapy in the third trimester in HBV-infected pregnant women to further reduce the risk of MTCT *(157, 472, 473)*.

Hepatitis C infection. Although the risk of MTCT of HCV infection is much lower than that of HBV infection, perinatal transmission of HCV occurs in between 4% and 8% of births, but the risk is two to three times higher if the mother is coinfected with HIV *(96)*. Although the costs of implementing HCV testing alongside HIV and HBV is likely to be low, there is currently no effective public health intervention to decrease the risk of MTCT of HCV infection. However, identifying pregnant women who are HCV positive allows avoidance of procedures that promote mixing of fetal and maternal blood (e.g. use of scalp electrodes, amniocentesis), and may thus decrease transmission risk *(98)*. It can also help promote testing of the child at 18 months. Identifying and treating women of reproductive age before they become pregnant preferable, but if DAAs are found to be safe and effective for use in pregnancy, they will also contribute to the prevention of MTCT.

Implementation considerations

- **Integration with HIV testing.** WHO now recommends HIV testing for all pregnant women *(11)*. The offer of HBV testing alongside existing HIV testing and PMTCT interventions is an effective and efficient mechanism of scaling up HBV testing for pregnant women and their partners. Information on risk factors for HCV infection should be communicated to pregnant women and, if present, or in high-endemic settings, testing for HCV should also be considered alongside testing for HIV and HBV.

- **Timing of testing.** Testing should be done as early as possible during pregnancy to enable pregnant women to benefit most from prevention, treatment and care, and to reduce the risk of transmission to their infants. It can also be performed late in pregnancy, in labour or, if that is not feasible, as soon as possible after delivery.

- **Pre- and post-test counselling.** Pre-test information for women who are or may become pregnant or who are postpartum should include: the benefits of early diagnosis of HBV or HCV infection for their own health, as well as to reduce the risk of HBV or HCV transmission to the infant; and importance of testing also for HIV and syphilis. Post-test counselling should include: use of antiviral therapy for the mother's health as appropriate; measures to reduce the risk of transmitting HBV or HCV infection to the infant; encouragement for partner testing; advice on childbirth plans and infant-feeding options with an encouragement to deliver in a health facility to ensure access to PMTCT services; and HBV and HCV testing for the infant.

- **Linkage to care.** There is a significant loss to follow up of pregnant women testing HBV- or HCV-positive who need to be linked to care to assess the need for antiviral treatment and ongoing monitoring. Pregnant women without any serological markers for HBV can be offered HBV vaccination. Follow up should continue through the breastfeeding period to ensure that infants born to mothers with CHB receive the recommended three doses of vaccine, especially if they did not receive the HBV birth-dose vaccination.

18.9. Children

There are significant gaps and missed opportunities for diagnosis and documenting the HBV and HCV status of children of HBV-positive parents or HCV-positive mothers.

Hepatitis B infection. In endemic countries, HBV- infection is predominantly transmitted perinatally or in early childhood. In some settings, up to 50% of childhood infections may be attributable to horizontal intrafamilial transmission. In non-endemic settings, most children with CHB are migrants or children of migrants from endemic countries. Box 18.1 summarizes the existing WHO guidelines on HBV infection prevention in newborns. Although 70–90% of children who are exposed perinatally will become chronically infected, HBV-related morbidity is low during childhood as they are generally in the immune-tolerant phase. Since there are also low curative rates with both long-term NA and IFN treatment, and concerns over long-term safety and risk of drug resistance, a conservative approach to antiviral therapy is indicated, unless there are other criteria for treatment, such as cirrhosis or evidence of severe ongoing necroinflammatory disease *(6)*. Tenofovir is approved for use in adolescents and children above the age of 12 years for HBV treatment (and 3 years or older for HIV treatment), and entecavir above 2 years of age.

> **Box 18.1. WHO recommendations on HBV prevention in newborns and children**
>
> All infants should receive their first dose of hepatitis B vaccine as soon as possible after birth, preferably within 24 hours, followed by two or three doses.
>
> HBIG prophylaxis, in conjunction with HBV vaccination, may be of additional benefit for the following: newborn infants whose mothers are HBsAg positive, particularly if they are also HBeAg positive. In full-term neonates born to mothers who are HBsAg positive but HBeAg negative, protection against perinatally acquired infection achieved by immediate vaccination against HBV (given within 24 hours) may not be significantly improved by the addition of HBIG.
>
> *Source:* Guidelines for the prevention, care and treatment of persons with chronic hepatitis B infection. Geneva: WHO; 2015 ((http://apps.who.int/iris/bitstream/10665/154590/1/9789241549059_eng.pdf?ua=1&ua=1) *(6)*.

Hepatitis C infection. In countries where adults have a high prevalence of HCV infection, an increased prevalence in children is often observed. This rate is particularly high in those exposed to medical interventions and treated in hospitals *(101)*. Children born to mothers with HCV infection, especially those who are HIV-coinfected, are also at risk *(96–99)*, and MTCT is the most common cause of HCV infection in young children.

As with HBV infection, the progression of HCV liver disease is usually slow in infected children. None of the DAAs have yet been approved for use among children (data from ongoing clinical trials will provide the necessary safety and efficacy data for paediatric regulatory approval), and so the only approved treatment remains PEG-IFN/ribavirin. However, as DAAs offer the potential for curative treatment at an early stage before progression of liver disease in children, earlier HCV testing in infants and children will also become more important.

Implementation considerations

- **Service delivery approaches to delivering testing to infants and children.** Box 18.2 shows potential testing approaches to improve hepatitis case-finding among infants and children. Infants whose mothers have been diagnosed with HBV or HCV should be followed up and routinely offered testing, and those diagnosed with either should be regularly monitored for signs of liver disease so that treatment can be offered when necessary. In high-prevalence settings, testing of HBV- and HCV-exposed infants could be available through a variety of services – child health services, immunization clinics, under-5 clinics, malnutrition services, well-child services, services for hospitalized and all sick children, TB clinics, and services for orphans and vulnerable children. Follow up through the breastfeeding period is also important to be able to offer HBV testing and vaccination for infants born to mothers with CHB who did not receive the HBV birth-dose vaccination, and to ensure that all children are followed up to receive the recommended three doses of vaccine. However, many infants are lost to follow up, which makes additional paediatric case-finding important.

- **Testing in infants and children under 18 months. Hepatitis B.** Testing of exposed infants is problematic within the first six months of life, as HBsAg and HBV DNA may be inconsistently detectable in infected infants. Exposed infants should be tested for HBsAg at 12 months of age – CHB is diagnosed if there is persistence of HBsAg for six months or more *(95)*. **Hepatitis C.** HCV infection in children under 18 months can be confirmed only by virological assays to detect HCV RNA, because transplacental maternal antibodies remain in the child's bloodstream up until 18 months of age, making test results from serology assays ambiguous.

> **Box 18.2 Potential testing approaches to improve hepatitis case-finding among infants and children**
>
> - Prioritize testing children of all HBV- or HCV-positive mothers (especially if the mother is HCV/HIV-coinfected) through home- or facility-based testing.
> - Offer testing to all children and adolescents presenting with signs and symptoms that suggest acute viral hepatitis, including anorexia, nausea, jaundice, right upper quadrant discomfort and abnormal liver function tests.
> - Consider offering viral hepatitis testing to all children and adolescents attending HIV services, STI clinics and TB clinics.
> - Offer viral hepatitis testing or retesting to mothers or infants in immunization clinics or under-5 clinics.
> - Target HCV testing to children who have had medical interventions or received blood products in countries where screening of blood is not routine or where medical equipment is inadequately sterilized.

18.10. Adolescents

In high HBV- or HCV-prevalence settings, two groups of adolescents (defined as 10–19 years of age) are at potential risk of HBV or HCV infection and may need access to testing. These include the following: (1) **undiagnosed adolescents who were HBV exposed perinatally or in early childhood** in highly endemic HBV settings, and who missed out on HBV vaccination. These adolescents need to be diagnosed and started on antiviral treatment if and when this is clinically indicated, or if negative, vaccinated for HBV. (2) **Adolescents who acquire HBV or HCV sexually or through injecting drug use** through sex with multiple partners, or with MSM. It is important that these adolescents receive targeted interventions to increase access to HIV and hepatitis testing *(474)*.

Implementation considerations

- **Service delivery – delivering adolescent-friendly services.** Engaging adolescents in testing for both HIV and viral hepatitis, either within the health services or community, should be based on adolescent-friendly principles to ensure that psychological as well as physical needs are addressed. Services need to be convenient and available, offer flexible opening hours and/or walk-in or same-day appointments. Separate hours and special events for adolescents may help overcome concerns that they will be seen attending viral hepatitis/HIV services by relatives or neighbours.

- **Disclosure.** Adolescents may particularly need support with when and to whom to disclose a positive status *(474)*. When appropriate, and only with the adolescent's specific permission, health-care personnel should engage the support of adults – family members, teachers, community members.

- **Vulnerable adolescents.** Special considerations are needed for particularly vulnerable adolescents, such as those living on the streets, orphans, boys who have sex with men, adolescents in child-headed households, girls engaged in sex with older men, in multiple or concurrent sexual partnerships, or those who are sexually exploited *(25)*. Specific campaigns, use of social media or other web-based approaches, and involving adolescents in identifying appropriate language may help to reach this group in some settings.

- **Age of consent.** The age of consent for HIV testing varies from country to country, and this can pose barriers to adolescents' access to HIV and viral hepatitis testing *(474)*. Testing services should be aware of laws and policies governing the age of consent, and develop appropriate procedures based on this legal framework to ensure that children and adolescents have access to testing. WHO also recommends that children and adolescents themselves be involved in the testing decision as much as possible *(474)*.

Further reading

HIV and adolescents: guidance for HIV testing and counselling and care for adolescents living with HIV. Geneva: WHO; 2013 *(474)*.

19. STRATEGIC PLANNING FOR IMPLEMENTING TESTING SERVICES AND APPROACHES

This chapter provides a strategic framework to guide countries' decision-making on selecting testing approaches, and summarizes the key steps for assessing and improving the selection of hepatitis testing approaches. This includes setting targets, reviewing the effectiveness of existing testing activities and identifying gaps, and then adjusting programme activities.

Key points

- There are many facility- and community-based opportunities for and approaches to delivering viral hepatitis testing (*see* Chapter 17). Countries need to consider a strategic mix of these testing approaches to reach different populations, identify people who are unaware that they are infected in the early stages of infection, and support the timely linkage to prevention, care and treatment services for those who test positive or negative.

- The selection and mix of testing approaches and application of effective programming practices should be based on a situational assessment that includes: national context and epidemiology (prevalence, populations affected and undiagnosed burden); existing health-care and testing infrastructure; current testing uptake and coverage (number and proportion ever tested by population); programme costs and cost–effectiveness of different testing approaches at national and subnational levels; available financial and human resources; and preferences of the populations to be served.

- All available epidemiological data from surveillance, surveys and programmes should be used to guide geographical, population, facility and service prioritization.

- Programmes should monitor data from testing services and in general favour the testing approaches that result in the highest proportion of positive diagnoses in priority populations.

Key steps for assessing and selecting hepatitis testing approaches

Box 19.1 and Fig. 19.1 summarize the key steps for assessing and improving the selection of hepatitis testing approaches, which include setting targets, reviewing the effectiveness of existing testing activities and identifying gaps, and then adjusting programme activities.

The final selection and mix of testing approaches with the greatest public health benefit and impact should be based on a situational assessment. This assessment should consider prevalence, unmet need (the estimated number of people who remain undiagnosed), priority populations for the country and the anticipated proportion testing positive, gaps in coverage in geographical areas with undiagnosed HBV and/or HCV infection, the available financial and human resources, and cost–effectiveness. Overall, a mix of hepatitis testing approaches that are focused on populations and/or geographical locations with high HBV or HCV prevalence, and that maximize linkage will have the greatest impact and likely be most cost–effective.

FIG. 19.1. Steps to assess, select and evaluate hepatitis testing approaches

Set targets
Based on:
- Treatment targets
- Epidemiology
- Current coverage

Review effectiveness and identify gaps
- Proportion HBV- or HCV-positive by different testing approaches
- Cost per new case identified
- Linkage rate
- By population group and locale

Adjust programme
Identify areas for focus/re-focus
- Population
- Geography
- Sites and setting
- Clinical services and conditions

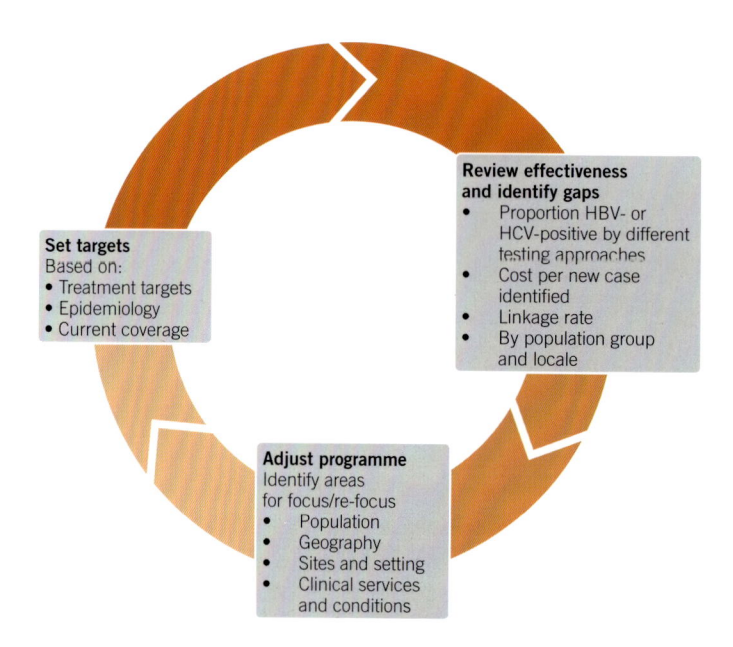

Box 19.1. Key steps for assessing and selecting hepatitis testing approaches

1. **Review national and subnational epidemiology** (prevalence, populations most affected and undiagnosed burden).

2. **Set testing (and treatment) coverage targets**.

3. **Review the effectiveness of existing testing services, and identify gaps.**
   This involves the following:
   - **mapping current services,** including availability, uptake (by sex, age and population), coverage rate, funding source and location of all current testing settings and sites;
   - **analysing data from the testing services** to assess current testing activities and coverage using different approaches in various sites and locations (e.g. number and proportion of people tested by population, age and sex, new cases diagnosed and enrolled in care);
   - **analysing and identifying gaps in current testing coverage** in relation to burden, by geographical location and population, focusing on areas of highest prevalence or incidence, which are not being reached by available services;
   - **assessing barriers to testing**, including social, cultural and geographical factors, psychosocial and behavioural factors, stigma and discrimination, gender and legal factors (including age-of-consent requirements), and structural and health system factors that may impede access;
   - **assessing linkage between testing and existing care and treatment programmes** following a positive diagnosis;
   - **assessing commodity and human resource needs;**
   - **assessing available human and financial resources**.

4. **Assess costs and cost–effectiveness of different testing approaches.**

5. **Monitor, evaluate and adjust testing programme activities.**

Step 1: Review national and subnational epidemiology

In order to devise successful testing services, it is important for countries to understand which populations and settings have the highest prevalence and incidence of HBV and HCV, the estimated number of people affected in the population, and where the greatest burden of undiagnosed infection exists geographically, and by age, sex and population group.

Although it is difficult to know the exact number of people with chronic hepatitis B or C infection or the number of new infections in a given area, this can be estimated through the analysis of all available epidemiological data from multiple sources, including surveillance, surveys and programmes. As population-based household surveys seldom reach or identify high-risk populations and marginalized vulnerable groups, additional studies may be required.

A summary of the epidemiological situation would include the following, and the information collated can be summarized in Table 19.1.

- **Estimates of HBsAg and HCV antibody prevalence in the general and specific high-risk populations**
    - **An estimate of HBsAg and HCV antibody prevalence in the general population** stratified by place (if relevant and available) and age group (for general population to identify which ages are at highest risk), as well as in pregnant women attending ANC from national population-based household surveys and surveillance data among pregnant women;
    - **For each high-risk population group** identified with a higher prevalence:
        - the prevalence of chronic infection in that population group
        - an estimation of the proportion of the infected population that belongs to that population group
        - an estimation of the size of that population group.

    Once the information on the prevalence has been summarized for the general population and specific groups, an analysis of the situation may guide the selection of groups to target with testing services. Testing population groups with a higher prevalence may have a higher yield but lead to the identification of a lower proportion of those living with infection. Testing the general population (or a defined age or birth cohort) may have a lower yield but leads to the identification of a larger proportion of those living with infection.

- **Hepatitis testing uptake**, by different populations and testing approaches;

and proportion of those tested who are positive, by population, testing approach or facility;

- **Number and proportion of people who are aware of their HBV and HCV status**
Depending on the data available, this may be the proportion of individuals who have ever been tested for HBV or HCV, or of people who were tested in the past 12 months and received their results. These data may be disaggregated by sex, age, geographical region, population type, testing approach and facility.

- **Proportion of people who tested positive and who have been enrolled in hepatitis care and treatment services.**

Step 2: Set testing (and treatment) coverage targets

For each type of testing service, a target may be set in terms of the number of persons to test and to refer for care and treatment or prevention if they are not infected but are at high ongoing risk. An additional target may include the proportion of persons living with viral hepatitis who are diagnosed. The consolidation of targets of all services considered will lead to an overall target for the number of persons for testing and treatment.

Coordinating testing with treatment scale up. As the primary reason for diagnosing people with chronic hepatitis B and C is so that they can benefit from treatment, it is important to directly link testing and treatment targets. Plans for major scale up of treatment services will not succeed without testing. Similarly, major scale up of testing, which will create a demand for treatment, will have limited benefit without concurrently expanding treatment capacity.

Step 3: Review the effectiveness of existing testing services and identify gaps

Following an epidemiological analysis, an assessment and mapping of current hepatitis testing activities and coverage can determine how well existing services are covering populations in need. This exercise could include the following and the information can be summarized in Table 19.1.

- **Mapping of existing services,** including location of all current testing settings and sites, uptake and coverage rate (by sex, age and population), and funding source. This may include facility-based testing in ANC, TB, STI clinics as well as in harm reduction, outpatient and inpatient services; outreach testing for key populations, community-based and mobile testing, testing within the workplace or educational institutions; and testing by private health-care providers.

A detailed situational assessment should also be undertaken with regard to HIV testing services, as in many settings the same populations may be affected, providing the opportunity to integrate hepatitis testing into existing HIV testing delivery models.

- **Analysing hepatitis testing services data** to see what is being achieved by specific approaches in various sites and locations, in terms of the number and proportion of people tested, new cases diagnosed and enrolled in care;

- **Analysing and identifying gaps in current hepatitis testing coverage** in relation to burden, by geographical location and population, focusing on areas of highest prevalence or incidence, which are not being reached by available services;

- **Assessing the strengths and weaknesses of these testing services, including preferences for testing approaches** through key informant interviews with clients and health-care workers;

- **Assessing barriers to testing,** including social, cultural and geographical factors, psychosocial and behavioural factors, stigma and discrimination, gender and legal factors (including age-of-consent requirements), and structural and health system factors that may impede access;

- **Assessing the linkage between hepatitis testing and existing care** and treatment programmes, in particular, following a positive diagnosis;

- **Assessing laboratory site performance**, including the quality of test performance;

- **Assessing commodity and human resource needs**, their availability, and policies to identify barriers to and opportunities for expanding or shifting the focus of programmes (e.g. availability of rapid test kits or trained lay providers and policies regarding task-sharing), and what education, training and certification are required for those conducting tests. The initial assessment should be followed by an inventory of the resources needed and available for testing services. These include (i) equipment (e.g. testing devices) and supplies (e.g. testing kits); (ii) financial resources; and (iii) human resources.

- **Assessing available financial resources for hepatitis testing,** including investments by the government and funding partners.

Step 4: Assess costs and cost–effectiveness of different testing approaches

• **Assessing costs.** Comparing the costs associated with a given testing approach between countries can be challenging. Costs for similar services often differ significantly between countries and by testing approach within a country, due to both general cost differences between countries and to differences in the specific services provided (e.g. referral to a clinic for those testing positive versus enhanced linkage support), cadre of staff employed (e.g. nurses versus community health workers), and the ease of reaching different populations. Direct cost comparisons of different testing approaches are easier to interpret when they use the same costing inputs. A common approach to estimating costs involves identifying costs incurred in the following broad categories: personnel (e.g. staff salaries and allowances); recurrent costs (e.g. test kits and commodities, printed materials, office supplies); and capital expenses, often totalled over their useful life and discounted annually at 3% (e.g. office space, vehicles, equipment). These costs can be added to compute the total expected cost of an intervention per year.

• **Estimating cost–effectiveness.** Cost–effectiveness analyses compare the costs and health impacts of different interventions to identify those that provide good value for money, and are useful for optimizing the allocation of public health resources. Health outcomes used in cost–effectiveness analyses of hepatitis testing services include: number of people tested; number of hepatitis B or C cases identified; number of infections averted (when linked to vaccination and prevention of MTCT); number of disability-adjusted life-years (DALYs) lost or number of quality-adjusted life-years (QALYs) gained (dependent not only on being diagnosed but linked to treatment).

The health benefits associated with testing are not derived from the test itself, but rather from the treatment and prevention interventions that occur subsequently, including the effectiveness of linkage from testing to treatment. The cost of a programme and its relative cost–effectiveness also depends greatly on the specifics of the programme itself. For example, a programme designed to reach PWID by running mobile camps at various locations can have significantly different costs from providing testing in a fixed location, such as a drug treatment programme. Still, both testing approaches may be necessary to reach this key population. Assessing which testing approaches make the most efficient use of resources requires a detailed understanding of the approaches themselves, including how and to whom they are delivered. Different approaches may be cost–effective for different populations.

Step 5: Monitor, evaluate and adjust programme activities

Ensuring that hepatitis testing programmes are reaching their intended populations and identifying previously undiagnosed positive persons will require continued monitoring and evaluation. For long-term success, the impact of different hepatitis testing approaches on uptake, the proportion that tests positive, costs, and changes in the prevalence of hepatitis B or C in different population groups must be evaluated and measured regularly, and programmes must be adjusted appropriately. Other activities include the following:

- Revisit and revise national targets for and approaches to hepatitis testing so as to better reach those who are undiagnosed, taking into account linkage and enrolment in treatment.

- Develop and follow a national consensus plan for expanding and refocusing hepatitis testing in line with the treatment plan.

- Evaluate implemented programmes through routine programme monitoring, programme-specific evaluations, surveillance and population-based surveys.

- Testing services also require their own monitoring and evaluation framework. In 2016, WHO published a monitoring and evaluation framework for hepatitis B and C (*Monitoring and evaluation for viral hepatitis B and C: recommended indicators and framework.* Geneva: WHO, 2016) that proposes ten core indicators *(22)*, and includes the proportion of persons living with HBV or HCV infection diagnosed.

Table 19.1. A simplified sample template of results of a baseline assessment of testing services

Examples of populations	Prevalence of infection in the group	Proportion of population with the characteristic	Estimated size of population	Estimated proportion of infected population that belongs to the population group	Number of tests conducted annually	Proportion of the population that is aware of its status	Facility or community service access points – Access point	Strengths	Weaknesses
General population	XX%	100%	XXXXXX	100%	XXXX	XX%	Primary care		
							Hospital		
Pregnant women	XX%	XX%	XXXXXX	XX%	XXXX	XX%	ANC clinics		
PWID	XX%	XX%	XXXXXX	XX%	XXXX	XX%	OST services		
MSM	XX%	XX%	XXXXXX	XX%	XXXX	XX%	Outreach		
Persons undergoing haemodialysis	XX%	XX%	XXXXXX	XX%	XXXX	XX%	Dialysis centres		

REFERENCES

1. GBD 2013 Mortality and Causes of Death Collaborators. Global, regional, and national age-sex specific all-cause and cause-specific mortality for 240 causes of death, 1990–2013: a systematic analysis for the Global Burden of Disease Study 2013. Lancet. 2015;385(9963):117–71.
2. Schweitzer A, Horn J, Mikolajczyk RT, Krause G, Ott JJ. Estimations of worldwide prevalence of chronic hepatitis B virus infection: a systematic review of data published between 1965 and 2013. Lancet. 2015;386(10003):1546–55.
3. Gower E, Estes C, Blach S, Razavi-Shearer K, Razavi H. Global epidemiology and genotype distribution of the hepatitis C virus infection. J Hepatol. 2014;61(1 Suppl):S45–S57.
4. Schinazi R, Halfon P, Marcellin P, Asselah T. HCV direct-acting antiviral agents: the best interferon-free combinations. Liver Int. 2014;34 Suppl 1:69–78.
5. Guidelines for the screening, care and treatment of persons with chronic hepatitis C infection. Updated version, April 2016. Geneva: World Health Organization; 2016 (http://apps.who.int/iris/bitstream/10665/205035/1/9789241549615_eng.pdf?ua=1, accessed 6 February 2017).
6. Guidelines for the prevention, care and treatment of persons with chronic hepatitis B infection. Geneva: World Health Organization; 2015 (http://apps.who.int/iris/bitstream/10665/154590/1/9789241549059_eng.pdf?ua=1&ua=1, 6 February 2017).
7. Mathurin P. HCV burden in Europe and the possible impact of current treatment. Dig Liver Dis. 2013;45(Suppl 5):S314–S317.
8. Mitchell AE, Colvin HM, Palmer Beasley R. Institute of Medicine recommendations for the prevention and control of hepatitis B and C. Hepatology. 2010;51(3):729–33.
9. Papatheodoridis G, Sypsa V, Kantzanou M, Nikolakopoulos I, Hatzakis A. Estimating the treatment cascade of chronic hepatitis B and C in Greece using a telephone survey. J Viral Hepat. 2015;22(4):409–15.
10. Hatzakis A, Wait S, Bruix J, Buti M, Carballo M, Cavaleri M et al. The state of hepatitis B and C in Europe: report from the hepatitis B and C summit conference. J Viral Hepat. 2011;18 (Suppl 1):1–16.
11. Consolidated guidelines on HIV testing services. Geneva: World Health Organization; 2015 (http://apps.who.int/iris/bitstream/10665/179870/1/9789241508926_eng.pdf?ua=1&ua=1, 6 February 2017).
12. Technical considerations and case definitions to improve surveillance for viral hepatitis. Geneva: World Health Organization; 2016 (http://www.who.int/hepatitis/publications/hep-surveillance-guide-pub/en/, accessed 6 February 2017).
13. Resolution WHA63.18. Viral hepatitis. In: Sixty-third World Health Assembly. Geneva: World Health Organization; 2010 (http://apps.who.int/gb/ebwha/pdf_files/WHA63-REC1/WHA63_REC1-en.pdf accessed 6 February 2017).
14. Resolution WHA67.6. Hepatitis. In: Sixty-seventh World Health Assembly. Geneva: World Health Organization; 2014 (http://apps.who.int/gb/ebwha/pdf_files/WHA67/A67_R6-en.pdf accessed 6 February 2017).
15. Guidelines for the screening, care and treatment of persons with hepatitis C infection. Geneva: World Health Organization; 2014 (http://apps.who.int/iris/bitstream/10665/111747/1/9789241548755_eng.pdf?ua=1&ua=1, accessed 6 February 2017).
16. WHO global health sector strategy on viral hepatitis. Geneva: World Health Organization; 2016 (http://www.who.int/hepatitis/strategy2016-2021/Draft_global_health_sector_strategy_viral_hepatitis_13nov.pdf?ua=1, accessed 16 February 2017).
17. Hepatitis A. Fact sheet. Geneva: World Health Organization; July 2016 (http://www.who.int/mediacentre/factsheets/fs328/en/, accessed 05 February 2017).
18. Waterborne outbreaks of hepatitis E: recognition, investigation and control. Geneva: World Health Organization; 2014 (http://apps.who.int/iris/bitstream/10665/129448/1/9789241507608_eng.pdf?ua=1&ua=1, accessed 6 February 2017).
19. Hepatitis delta. Fact sheet. Geneva: World Health Organization; July 2016 (http://www.who.int/mediacentre/factsheets/hepatitis-d/en/, 05 February 2017).
20. Screening donated blood for transfusion transmissible infections. Geneva: World Health Organization; 2010 (http://www.who.int/bloodsafety/ScreeningDonatedBloodforTransfusion.pdf, accessed 6 February 2017).
21. HIV self-testing and partner notification. Geneva: World Health Organization; 2016 (http://apps.who.int/iris/bitstream/10665/251655/1/9789241549868-eng.pdf?ua=1, accessed 19 January 2017).
22. Monitoring and evaluation for viral hepatitis B and C: recommended indicators and framework: technical report. Geneva: World Health Organization; 2016 (http://apps.who.int/iris/bitstream/10665/204790/1/9789241510288_eng.pdf, accessed 6 February 2017).
23. Consolidated guidelines on the use of antiretrovirals for treating and preventing HIV infection. Recommendations for a public health approach. Geneva: World Health Organization; 2016 (http://apps.who.int/iris/bitstream/10665/208825/1/9789241549684_eng.pdf?ua=1, accessed 6 February 2017).
24. Hepatitis B vaccines. Wkly Epidemiol Rec. 2009;84:405–20.
25. Consolidated guidelines on HIV prevention, diagnosis, treatment and care for key populations. Geneva: World Health Organization; 2014 (http://apps.who.int/iris/bitstream/10665/128048/1/9789241507431_eng.pdf?ua=1&ua=1, accessed 6 February 2017).

26. Prevention and treatment of HIV and other sexually transmitted infections among men who have sex with men and transgender people. Geneva: World Health Organization; 2011 (http://apps.who.int/iris/bitstream/10665/44619/1/9789241501750_eng.pdf, accessed 6 February 2017).
27. Prevention and treatment of HIV and other sexually transmitted infections for sex workers in low- and middle-income countries: recommendations for a public health approach. Geneva: World Health Organization; 2012 (https://www.unfpa.org/sites/default/files/pub-pdf/9789241504744_eng.pdf, accessed 6 February 2017).
28. Guidance on prevention of viral hepatitis B and C among people who inject drugs. Geneva: World Health Organization; 2012 (http://apps.who.int/iris/bitstream/10665/75357/1/9789241504041_eng.pdf?ua=1, accessed 18 December 2016).
29. WHO guidelines on hand hygiene in health care. Geneva: World Health Organization; 2009 (http://apps.who.int/iris/bitstream/10665/44102/1/9789241597906_eng.pdf, accessed 6 February 2017).
30. Universal access to safe blood transfusion. Geneva: World Health Organization; 2008 (http://www.who.int/bloodsafety/publications/UniversalAccesstoSafeBT.pdf?ua=1, accessed 6 February 2017).
31. WHO guideline on the use of safety-engineered syringes for intramuscular, intradermal and subcutaneous injections in health care settings. Geneva: World Health Organization; 2016.
32. The Universal Declaration of Human Rights. Geneva: United Nations; 1948 (http://www.un.org/en/documents/udhr/index.shtml, accessed 6 February 2017).
33. Handbook for guideline development, second edition. Geneva: World Health Organization; 2014 (http://apps.who.int/iris/bitstream/10665/145714/1/9789241548960_eng.pdf, accessed 6 February 2017).
34. Guyatt G, Oxman AD, Akl EA, Kunz R, Vist G, Brozek J et al. GRADE guidelines: 1. Introduction – GRADE evidence profiles and summary of findings tables. J Clin Epidemiol. 2011;64(4):383–94.
35. Balshem H, Helfand M, Schunemann HJ, Oxman AD, Kunz R, Brozek J et al. GRADE guidelines: 3. Rating the quality of evidence. J Clin Epidemiol. 2011;64(4):401–6.
36. Guyatt GH, Oxman AD, Kunz R, Atkins D, Brozek J, Vist G et al. GRADE guidelines: 2. Framing the question and deciding on important outcomes. J Clin Epidemiol. 2011;64(4):395–400.
37. Andrews J, Guyatt G, Oxman AD, Alderson P, Dahm P, Falck-Ytter Y et al. GRADE guidelines: 14. Going from evidence to recommendations: the significance and presentation of recommendations. J Clin Epidemiol. 2013;66(7):719–25.
38. Schunemann HJ, Oxman AD, Brozek J, Glasziou P, Jaeschke R, Vist GE et al. Grading quality of evidence and strength of recommendations for diagnostic tests and strategies. BMJ. 2008;336(7653):1106–10.
39. Gopalakrishna G, Mustafa RA, Davenport C, Scholten RJ, Hyde C, Brozek J et al. Applying Grading of Recommendations Assessment, Development and Evaluation (GRADE) to diagnostic tests was challenging but doable. J Clin Epidemiol. 2014;67(7):760–8.
40. Whiting PF, Rutjes AW, Westwood ME, Mallett S, Deeks JJ, Reitsma JB et al. QUADAS-2: a revised tool for the quality assessment of diagnostic accuracy studies. Ann Intern Med. 2011;155(8):529–36.
41. Guyatt GH, Oxman AD, Vist G, Kunz R, Brozek J, Alonso-Coello P et al. GRADE guidelines: 4. Rating the quality of evidence--study limitations (risk of bias). J Clin Epidemiol. 2011;64(4):407–15.
42. Guyatt GH, Oxman AD, Montori V, Vist G, Kunz R, Brozek J et al. GRADE guidelines: 5. Rating the quality of evidence – publication bias. J Clin Epidemiol. 2011;64(12):1277–82.
43. Guyatt GH, Oxman AD, Kunz R, Brozek J, Alonso-Coello P, Rind D et al. GRADE guidelines 6. Rating the quality of evidence – imprecision. J Clin Epidemiol. 2011;64(12):1283–93.
44. Guyatt GH, Oxman AD, Kunz R, Woodcock J, Brozek J, Helfand M et al. GRADE guidelines: 7. Rating the quality of evidence – inconsistency. J Clin Epidemiol. 2011;64(12):1294–302.
45. Guyatt GH, Oxman AD, Kunz R, Woodcock J, Brozek J, Helfand M et al. GRADE guidelines: 8. Rating the quality of evidence – indirectness. J Clin Epidemiol. 2011;64(12):1303–10.
46. Nelson PK, Mathers BM, Cowie B, Hagan H, Des Jarlais D, Horyniak D et al. Global epidemiology of hepatitis B and hepatitis C in people who inject drugs: results of systematic reviews. Lancet. 2011;378(9791):571–83.
47. Lok AS, McMahon BJ. Chronic hepatitis B. Hepatology. 2007;45(2):507–39.
48. Scheinmann R, Hagan H, Lelutiu-Weinberger C, Stern R, Des Jarlais DC, Flom PL et al. Non-injection drug use and hepatitis C virus: a systematic review. Drug Alcohol Depen. 2007;89(1):1–12.
49. El Maerrawi I, Carvalho HB. Prevalence and risk factors associated with HIV infection, hepatitis and syphilis in a state prison of Sao Paulo. Int J STD AIDS. 2015;26(2):120–7.
50. Evidence for action technical papers: effectiveness of interventions to address HIV in prisons. Geneva: World Health Organization; 2007 (http://apps.who.int/iris/bitstream/10665/43806/1/9789241596190_eng.pdf, accessed 6 February 2017).
51. Larney S, Kopinski H, Beckwith CG, Zaller ND, Jarlais DD, Hagan H et al. Incidence and prevalence of hepatitis C in prisons and other closed settings: results of a systematic review and meta-analysis. Hepatology. 2013;58(4):1215–24.
52. Padovese V, Egidi AM, Melillo TF, Farrugia B, Carabot P, Didero D et al. Prevalence of latent tuberculosis, syphilis, hepatitis B and C among asylum seekers in Malta. J Public Health (Oxf). 2014;36(1):22–7.
53. Policy statement on HIV testing and counselling for refugees and other persons of concern to UNHCR. Geneva: United Nations High Commissioner for Refugees; 2014 (http://www.unhcr.org/53a816729.pdf, accessed 6 February 2017).

54. Hahne SJ, Veldhuijzen IK, Wiessing L, Lim TA, Salminen M, Laar M. Infection with hepatitis B and C virus in Europe: a systematic review of prevalence and cost-effectiveness of screening. BMC Infect Dis. 2013;13:181.
55. Bloodborne viral and sexually transmissible infections in Aboriginal and Torres Strait Islander people: annual surveillance report 2015. Sydney, Australia: The Kirby Institute for infection and immunity in society 2015 (https://kirby.unsw.edu.au/sites/default/files/hiv/resources/atsip2015_v3.pdf, accessed 8 February 2017).
56. Implementing comprehensive HIV/STI programmes with sex workers: practical approaches from collaborative interventions. Geneva: World Health Organization; 2013 (http://apps.who.int/iris/bitstream/10665/90000/1/9789241506182_eng.pdf, accessed 6 February 2017).
57. Policy brief: transgender people and HIV. Geneva: World Helath Organization; 2015 (http://apps.who.int/iris/bitstream/10665/179517/1/WHO_HIV_2015.17_eng.pdf?ua=1, accessed 5 February 2017).
58. Diamond C, Thiede H, Perdue T, Secura GM, Valleroy L, Mackellar D et al. Viral hepatitis among young men who have sex with men: prevalence of infection, risk behaviors, and vaccination. Sex Transm Dis. 2003;30(5):425–32.
59. Tohme RA, Holmberg SD. Is sexual contact a major mode of hepatitis C virus transmission? Hepatology. 2010;52(4):1497–505.
60. Yaphe S, Bozinoff N, Kyle R, Shivkumar S, Pai NP, Klein M. Incidence of acute hepatitis C virus infection among men who have sex with men with and without HIV infection: a systematic review. Sex Transm Infect. 2012;88(7):558–64.
61. Bradshaw D, Matthews G, Danta M. Sexually transmitted hepatitis C infection: the new epidemic in MSM? Curr Opin Infect Dis. 2013;26(1):66–72.
62. Rauch A, Rickenbach M, Weber R, Hirschel B, Tarr PE, Bucher HC et al. Unsafe sex and increased incidence of hepatitis C virus infection among HIV-infected men who have sex with men: The Swiss HIV cohort study. Clin Infect Dis. 2005;41(3):395–402.
63. van de Laar T, Pybus O, Bruisten S, Brown D, Nelson M, Bhagani S et al. Evidence of a large, international network of HCV transmission in HIV-positive men who have sex with men. Gastroenterology. 2009;136(5):1609–17.
64. Fierer DS, Uriel AJ, Carriero DC, Klepper A, Dieterich DT, Mullen MP et al. Liver fibrosis during an outbreak of acute hepatitis c virus infection in HIV-infected men: a prospective cohort study. J Infect Dis. 2008;198(5):683–6.
65. Danta M, Brown D, Bhagani S, Pybus OG, Sabin CA, Nelson M et al. Recent epidemic of acute hepatitis C virus in HIV-positive men who have sex with men linked to high-risk sexual behaviours. AIDS. 2007;21(8):983–91.
66. Deuffic-Burban S, Delarocque-Astagneau E, Abiteboul D, Bouvet E, Yazdanpanah Y. Blood-borne viruses in health care workers: prevention and management. J Clin Virol. 2011;52(1):4–10.
67. Lee R. Occupational transmission of bloodborne diseases to healthcare workers in developing countries: meeting the challenges. J Hosp Infect. 2009;72(4):285–91.
68. Beltrami EM, Williams IT, Shapiro CN, Chamberland ME. Risk and management of blood-borne infections in health care workers. Clin Microbiol Rev. 2000;13(3):385–407.
69. Global database on blood safety. In: Blood transfusion safety [webpage]. Geneva: World Health Organization; 2011 (http://www.who.int/bloodsafety/global_database/en/, accessed 6 February 2017).
70. Shepard CW, Finelli L, Alter MJ. Global epidemiology of hepatitis C virus infection. Lancet Int Dis. 2005;5(9).558–67.
71. Frank C, Mohamed MK, Strickland GT, Lavanchy D, Arthur RR, Magder LS et al. The role of parenteral antischistosomal therapy in the spread of hepatitis C virus in Egypt. Lancet. 2000;355(9207):887–91.
72. Singh S, Dwivedi SN, Sood R, Wali JP. Hepatitis B, C and human immunodeficiency virus infections in multiply-injected kala-azar patients in Delhi. Scand J Infect Dis. 2000;32(1):3–6.
73. Marx MA, Murugavel KG, Sivaram S, Balakrishnan P, Steinhoff M, Anand S et al. The association of health-care use and hepatitis C virus infection in a random sample of urban slum community residents in southern India. Am J Trop Med Hyg. 2003;68(2):258–62.
74. Wang CS, Chang TT, Chou P. Differences in risk factors for being either a hepatitis B carrier or anti-hepatitis C+ in a hepatoma-hyperendemic area in rural Taiwan. J Clin Epidemiol. 1998;51(9):733–8.
75. Ho MS, Hsu CP, Yuh Y, King CC, Tsai JF. High rate of hepatitis C virus infection in an isolated community: persistent hyperendemicity or period-related phenomena? J Med Virol. 1997;52(4):370–6.
76. Lin CC, Hwang SJ, Chiou ST, Kuan CL, Chen LW, Lee TC et al. The prevalence and risk factors analysis of serum antibody to hepatitis C virus in the elders in northeast Taiwan. J Chin Med Assoc. 2003;66(2):103–8.
77. Saxena R, Thakur V, Sood B, Guptan RC, Gururaja S, Sarin SK. Transfusion-associated hepatitis in a tertiary referral hospital in India. A prospective study. Vox Sang. 1999;77(1):6–10.
78. Candotti D, Sarkodie F, Allain JP. Residual risk of transfusion in Ghana. Br J Haematol. 2001;113(1):37–9.
79. Ministry of Health and Population [Egypt], El-Zanaty and Associates [Egypt], ICF International. Egypt Demographic and Health Survey 2014. Cairo, Egypt and Rockville, Maryland, USA: Ministry of Health and Population and ICF International; 2015.

80. Omar N, Salama K, Adolf S, El-Saeed GS, Abdel Ghaffar N, Ezzat N. Major risk of blood transfusion in hemolytic anemia patients. Blood Coagul Fibrinolysis. 2011;22(4):280–4.
81. Ghosh K, Joshi SH, Shetty S, Pawar A, Chipkar S, Pujari V et al. Transfusion transmitted diseases in haemophilics from western India. Indian J Med Res. 2000;112:61–4.
82. Arababadi MK, Nasiri Ahmadabadi B, Yousefi Daredor H, Kennedy D. Epidemiology of occult hepatitis B infection among thalassemic, hemophilia, and hemodialysis patients. Hepat Mon. 2012;12(5):315–9.
83. Nishioka Sde A, Gyorkos TW, Joseph L, Collet JP, Maclean JD. Tattooing and risk for transfusion-transmitted diseases: the role of the type, number and design of the tattoos, and the conditions in which they were performed. Epidemiol Infect. 2002;128(1):63–71.
84. Jafari S, Copes R, Baharlou S, Etminan M, Buxton J. Tattooing and the risk of transmission of hepatitis C: a systematic review and meta-analysis. Int J Infect Dis. 2010;14(11):E928–E940.
85. Karmochkine M, Carrat F, Dos Santos O, Cacoub P, Raguin G. A case control study of risk factors for hepatitis C infection in patients with unexplained routes of infection. J Viral Hepat. 2006;13(11):775–82.
86. Ezechi OC, Kalejaiye OO, Gab-Okafor CV, Oladele DA, Oke BO, Musa ZA et al. Sero-prevalence and factors associated with hepatitis B and C co-infection in pregnant Nigerian women living with HIV infection. Pan Afr Med J. 2014;17:197.
87. Easterbrook PJ, Platt L, Gower E, McDonald B, Sabin K, McGowan C et al. Global systematic review and meta-analysis of the seroprevalence of HBV and HCV infection in HIV-infected persons. 8th IAS Conference on HIV Pathogenesis, Treatment and Prevention. 19–22 July 2015. [Abstract No TU PEB254].
88. Platt L, Easterbrook P, Gower E, McDonald B, Sabin K, McGowan C et al. Prevalence and burden of HCV co-infection in people living with HIV: a global systematic review and meta-analysis. Lancet Infect Dis. 2016;16(7):797–808.
89. Karuru JW, Lule GN, Joshi M, Anzala O. Prevalence of HCV and HCV/HIV co-infection among in-patients at the Kenyatta National Hospital. East Afr Med J. 2005;82(4):170–2.
90. Quaranta JF, Delaney SR, Alleman S, Cassuto JP, Dellamonica P, Allain JP. Prevalence of antibody to hepatitis C virus (HCV) in HIV-1-infected patients (nice SEROCO cohort). J Med Virol. 1994;42(1):29–32.
91. Sherman KE, Rouster SD, Chung RT, Rajicic N. Hepatitis C virus prevalence among patients infected with human immunodeficiency virus: a cross-sectional analysis of the US adult AIDS Clinical Trials Group. Clin Infect Dis. 2002;34(6):831–7.
92. D'Oliveira A, Jr., Voirin N, Allard R, Peyramond D, Chidiac C, Touraine JL et al. Prevalence and sexual risk of hepatitis C virus infection when human immunodeficiency virus was acquired through sexual intercourse among patients of the Lyon University Hospitals, France, 1992–2002. J Viral Hepat. 2005;12(3):330–2.
93. Taylor LE, Swan T, Mayer KH. HIV coinfection with hepatitis C virus: evolving epidemiology and treatment paradigms. Clin Infect Dis. 2012;55 (Suppl 1):S33–S42.
94. Shimakawa Y, Toure-Kane C, Mendy M, Thursz M, Lemoine M. Mother-to-child transmission of hepatitis B in sub-Saharan Africa. Lancet Infect Dis. 2016;16(1):19–20.
95. McMahon BJ. The natural history of chronic hepatitis B virus infection. Semin Liver Dis. 2004;24 (Suppl 1):17–21.
96. Thomas DL, Villano SA, Riester KA, Hershow R, Mofenson LM, Landesman SH et al. Perinatal transmission of hepatitis C virus from human immunodeficiency virus type 1-infected mothers. Women and Infants Transmission Study. J Infect Dis. 1998;177(6):1480–8.
97. Benova L, Mohamoud YA, Calvert C, Abu-Raddad LJ. Vertical transmission of hepatitis C virus: systematic review and meta-analysis. Clin Infect Dis. 2014;59(6):765–73.
98. Mast EE, Hwang LY, Seto DS, Nolte FS, Nainan OV, Wurtzel H et al. Risk factors for perinatal transmission of hepatitis C virus (HCV) and the natural history of HCV infection acquired in infancy. J Infect Dis. 2005;192(11):1880–9.
99. Floreani A. Hepatitis C and pregnancy. World J Gastroenterol. 2013;19(40):6714–20.
100. Camarero C, Martos I, Delgado R, Suarez L, Escobar H, Mateos M. Horizontal transmission of hepatitis C virus in households of infected children. J Pediatr. 1993;123(1):98–9.
101. Thursz M, Fontanet A. HCV transmission in industrialized countries and resource-constrained areas. Nat Rev Gastroenterol Hepatol. 2014;11(1):28–35.
102. Terrault NA, Dodge JL, Murphy EL, Tavis JE, Kiss A, Levin TR et al. Sexual transmission of hepatitis C virus among monogamous heterosexual couples: the HCV partners study. Hepatology. 2013;57(3):881–9.
103. Gupta S, Gupta R, Joshi YK, Singh S. Role of horizontal transmission in hepatitis B virus spread among household contacts in north India. Intervirology. 2008;51(1):7–13.
104. Vandelli C, Renzo F, Romano L, Tisminetzky S, De Palma M, Stroffolini T et al. Lack of evidence of sexual transmission of hepatitis C among monogamous couples: results of a 10-year prospective follow-up study. Am J Gastroenterol. 2004;99(5):855–9.
105. Perz JF, Armstrong GL, Farrington LA, Hutin YJ, Bell BP. The contributions of hepatitis B virus and hepatitis C virus infections to cirrhosis and primary liver cancer worldwide. J Hepatol. 2006;45(4):529–38.
106. Goldstein ST, Zhou F, Hadler SC, Bell BP, Mast EE, Margolis HS. A mathematical model to estimate global hepatitis B disease burden and vaccination impact. Int J Epidemiol. 2005;34(6):1329–39.
107. Yi P, Chen R, Huang Y, Zhou RR, Fan XG. Management of mother-to-child transmission of hepatitis B virus: propositions and challenges. J Clin Virol. 2016;77:32–9.

108. Sarin SK, Kumar M, Lau GK, Abbas Z, Chan HL, Chen CJ et al. Asian-Pacific clinical practice guidelines on the management of hepatitis B: a 2015 update. Hepatol Int. 2016;10(1):1–98.
109. Lavanchy D. Hepatitis B virus epidemiology, disease burden, treatment, and current and emerging prevention and control measures. J Viral Hepat. 2004;11(2):97–107.
110. Yonghao G, Jin X, Jun L, Pumei D, Ying Y, Xiuhong F et al. An epidemiological serosurvey of hepatitis B virus shows evidence of declining prevalence due to hepatitis B vaccination in central China. Int J Infect Dis. 2015;40:75–80.
111. Wasley A, Kruszon-Moran D, Kuhnert W, Simard EP, Finelli L, McQuillan G et al. The prevalence of hepatitis B virus infection in the United States in the era of vaccination. J Infect Dis. 2010;202(2):192–201.
112. Head-to-head comparison of two years efficacy of entecavir and tenofovir in patients with treatment naive chronic hepatitis B – the real life data. Hepatogastroenterology. 2015;62(140):982–6.
113. Hadziyannis SJ. Update on hepatitis B virus infection: focus on treatment. J Clin Transl Hepatol. 2014;2(4):285–91.
114. Rao VB, Johari N, du Cros P, Messina J, Ford N, Cooke GS. Hepatitis C seroprevalence and HIV co-infection in sub-Saharan Africa: a systematic review and meta-analysis. Lancet Infect Dis. 2015;15(7):819–24.
115. Lozano R, Naghavi M, Foreman K, Lim S, Shibuya K, Aboyans V et al. Global and regional mortality from 235 causes of death for 20 age groups in 1990 and 2010: a systematic analysis for the Global Burden of Disease Study 2010. Lancet. 2012;380(9859):2095–128.
116. Razavi H, Waked I, Sarrazin C, Myers RP, Idilman R, Calinas F et al. The present and future disease burden of hepatitis C virus (HCV) infection with today's treatment paradigm. J Viral Hepat. 2014;21:34–59.
117. Eyster ME, Alter HJ, Aledort LM, Quan S, Hatzakis A, Goedert JJ. Heterosexual co-transmission of hepatitis C virus (HCV) and human immunodeficiency virus (HIV). Ann Intern Med. 1991;115(10):764–8.
118. Bica I, McGovern B, Dhar R, Stone D, McGowan K, Scheib R et al. Increasing mortality due to end-stage liver disease in patients with human immunodeficiency virus infection. Clin Infect Dis. 2001;32(3):492–7.
119. Ministry of Health and Population (Egypt), El-Zanaty and Associates (Egypt), ICF International. Egypt health issues survey 2015. Cairo, Egypt and Rockville, Maryland, USA: Ministry of Health and Population and ICF International; 2015.
120. Global database on blood safety. Summary report 2011. Geneva: World Health Organization; 2011 (http://www.who.int/bloodsafety/global_database/GDBS_Summary_Report_2011.pdf?ua=1, accessed 6 February 2017).
121. Marincovich B, Castilla J, del Romero J, Garcia S, Hernando V, Raposo M et al. Absence of hepatitis C virus transmission in a prospective cohort of heterosexual serodiscordant couples. Sex Transm Infect. 2003;79(2):160–2.
122. Tseng YT, Sun HY, Chang SY, Wu CH, Liu WC, Wu PY et al. Seroprevalence of hepatitis virus infection in men who have sex with men aged 18–40 years in Taiwan. J Formos Med Assoc. 2012;111(8):431–8.
123. Price H, Gilson R, Mercey D, Copas A, Parry J, Nardone A et al. Hepatitis C in men who have sex with men in London – a community survey. HIV Med. 2013;14(9):578–80.
124. Metwally A, Mohsen A, Saleh R, Foaud W, Ibrahim N, Rabaah T et al. Prioritizing high-risk practices and exploring new emerging ones associated with hepatitis C virus infection in Egypt. Iranian J Publ Health. 2014;43(10):1385–94.
125. Rein DB, Smith BD, Wittenborn JS, Lesesne SB, Wagner LD, Roblin DW et al. The cost-effectiveness of birth-cohort screening for hepatitis C antibody in US primary care settings. Ann Intern Med. 2012;156(4):263–70.
126. Mohd Hanafiah K, Groeger J, Flaxman AD, Wiersma ST. Global epidemiology of hepatitis C virus infection: new estimates of age-specific antibody to HCV seroprevalence. Hepatology. 2013;57(4):1333–42.
127. Alonso M, Gutzman A, Mazin R, Pinzon CE, Reveiz L, Ghidinelli M. Hepatitis C in key populations in Latin America and the Caribbean: systematic review and meta-analysis. Int J Public Health. 2015;60(7):789–98.
128. Chen Y, Shen Z, Morano JP, Khoshnood K, Wu Z, Lan G et al. Bridging the epidemic: a comprehensive analysis of prevalence and correlates of HIV, hepatitis C, and syphilis, and infection among female sex workers in Guangxi Province, China. PLoS One. 2015;10(2):e0115311.
129. Hagan H, Jordan AE, Neurer J, Cleland CM. Incidence of sexually transmitted hepatitis C virus infection in HIV-positive men who have sex with men. AIDS. 2015;29(17):2335–45.
130. Grebely J, Page K, Sacks-Davis R, van der Loeff MS, Rice TM, Bruneau J et al. The effects of female sex, viral genotype, and IL28B genotype on spontaneous clearance of acute hepatitis C virus infection. Hepatology. 2014;59(1):109–20.
131. Tong MJ, Elfarra NS, Reikes AR, Co RL. Clinical outcomes after transfusion-associated hepatitis-C. N Engl J Med. 1995;332(22):1463–6.
132. Tremolada F, Casarin C, Alberti A, Drago C, Tagger A, Ribero ML et al. Long-term follow-up of non-A, non-B (type C) post-transfusion hepatitis. J Hepatol. 1992;16(3):273–81.
133. Thein HH, Yi Q, Dore GJ, Krahn MD. Estimation of stage-specific fibrosis progression rates in chronic hepatitis C virus infection: a meta-analysis and meta-regression. Hepatology. 2008;48(2):418–31.

134. El-Serag HB, Rudolph KL. Hepatocellular carcinoma: epidemiology and molecular carcinogenesis. Gastroenterology. 2007;132(7):2557–76.

135. Busch MP. Insights into the epidemiology, natural history and pathogenesis of hepatitis C virus infection from studies of infected donors and blood product recipients. Transfus Clin Biol. 2001;8(3):200–6.

136. Abdelrahim SS, Khiry RM, Esmail MA, Ragab M, Abdel-Hamid M, Abdelwahab SF. Occult hepatitis C virus infection among Egyptian hemodialysis patients. J Med Virol. 2016;88(8):1388–93.

137. El-Shishtawy S, Sherif N, Abdallh E, Kamel L, Shemis M, Saleem AA et al. Occult hepatitis C virus infection in hemodialysis patients; single center study. Electron Physician. 2015;7(8):1619–25.

138. Rezaee-Zavareh MS, Hadi R, Karimi-Sari H, Hossein Khosravi M, Ajudani R, Dolatimehr F et al. Occult HCV infection: the current state of knowledge. Iran Red Crescent Med J. 2015;17(11):e34181.

139. Blood donor selection: guidelines on assessing donor suitability for blood donation. Geneva: World Health Organization; 2012 (http://www.ncbi.nlm.nih.gov/pubmed/23700651, accessed 6 February 2017).

140. WHO, UNODC, UNAIDS technical guide for countries to set targets for universal access to HIV prevention, treatment and care for injecting drug users. Geneva: World Health Organization; 2012 revision (http://apps.who.int/iris/bitstream/10665/77969/1/9789241504379_eng.pdf?ua=1, accessed 6 February 2017).

141. Allain JP, Opare-Sem O, Sarkodie F, Rahman R, Owusu-Ofori S. Deferred donor care in a regional hospital blood center in Ghana. Transfusion. 2009;49(4):669–75.

142. Pollack H, Wang S, Wyatt L, Peng CH, Wan K, Trinh-Shevrin C et al. A comprehensive screening and treatment model for reducing disparities in hepatitis B. Health Aff (Millwood). 2011;30(10):1974–83.

143. Eckman MH, Kaiser TE, Sherman KE. The cost-effectiveness of screening for chronic hepatitis B infection in the United States. Clin Infect Dis. 2011;52(11):1294–306.

144. Nayagam S, Conteh L, Sicuri E, Shimakawa Y, Suso P, Tamba S et al. Cost-effectiveness of community-based screening and treatment for chronic hepatitis B in The Gambia: an economic modelling analysis. Lancet Glob Health. 2016;4(8):e568–78.

145. Wong WW, Woo G, Jenny Heathcote E, Krahn M. Cost effectiveness of screening immigrants for hepatitis B. Liver Int. 2011;31(8):1179–90.

146. Rossi C, Schwartzman K, Oxlade O, Klein MB, Greenaway C. Hepatitis B screening and vaccination strategies for newly arrived adult Canadian immigrants and refugees: a cost-effectiveness analysis. PLoS One. 2013;8(10):e78548.

147. Hutton DW, Tan D, So SK, Brandeau ML. Cost-effectiveness of screening and vaccinating Asian and Pacific Islander adults for hepatitis B. Ann Intern Med. 2007;147(7):460–9.

148. Veldhuijzen IK, Toy M, Hahne SJ, De Wit GA, Schalm SW, de Man RA et al. Screening and early treatment of migrants for chronic hepatitis B virus infection is cost-effective. Gastroenterology. 2010;138(2):522–30.

149. Rein DB, Lesesne SB, Smith BD, Weinbaum CM. Models of community-based hepatitis B surface antigen screening programs in the US and their estimated outcomes and costs. Public Health Rep. 2011;126(4):560–7.

150. Jazwa A, Coleman MS, Gazmararian J, Wingate LT, Maskery B, Mitchell T et al. Cost-benefit comparison of two proposed overseas programs for reducing chronic Hepatitis B infection among refugees: is screening essential? Vaccine. 2015;33(11):1393–9.

151. Ruggeri M, Cicchetti A, Gasbarrini A. The cost-effectiveness of alternative strategies against HBV in Italy. Health Policy. 2011;102(1):72–80.

152. Lemoine M, Shimakawa Y, Nije R, Taal M, Ndow G, Chemin I et al., on behalf of the PROLIFICA investigators. Acceptability and feasibility of a screen-and-treat programme for hepatitis B virus infection in The Gambia: the Prevention of Liver Fibrosis and Cancer in Africa (PROLIFICA) study. Lancet Glob Health. 2016;4(8):e559–e567.

153. Easterbrook P, Johnson C, Figueroa C, Baggaley R. HIV and hepatitis testing: global progress, challenges and future directions. AIDS Rev. 2016;18:3–14.

154. Ott JJ, Stevens GA, Groeger J, Wiersma ST. Global epidemiology of hepatitis B virus infection: new estimates of age-specific HBsAg seroprevalence and endemicity. Vaccine. 2012;30(12):2212–9.

155. Qvist T, Cowan SA, Graugaard C, Helleberg M. High linkage to care in a community-based rapid HIV testing and counseling project among men who have sex with men in Copenhagen. Sex Transm Dis. 2014;41(3):209–14.

156. Hensen B, Baggaley R, Wong VJ, Grabbe KL, Shaffer N, Lo YR et al. Universal voluntary HIV testing in antenatal care settings: a review of the contribution of provider-initiated testing & counselling. Trop Med Int Health. 2012;17(1):59–70.

157. Thio CL, Guo N, Xie C, Nelson KE, Ehrhardt S. Global elimination of mother-to-child transmission of hepatitis B: revisiting the current strategy. Lancet Infect Dis. 2015;15(8):981–5.

158. Geue C, Wu O, Xin Y, Heggie R, Hutchinson S, Martin NK et al. Cost-effectiveness of HBV and HCV screening strategies – a systematic review of existing modelling techniques. PLoS One. 2015;10(12):e0145022.

159. Castelnuovo E, Thompson-Coon J, Pitt M, Cramp M, Siebert U, Price A et al. The cost-effectiveness of testing for hepatitis C in former injecting drug users. Health Technol Assess. 2006;10(32):iii–iv, ix–xii, 1–93.

160. Loubiere S, Rotily M, Moatti JP. Prevention could be less cost-effective than cure: the case of hepatitis C screening policies in France. Int J Technol Assess Health Care. 2003;19(4):632–45.
161. Loubiere S, Rotily M, Moatti JP. [Medico-economic assessment of the therapeutic management of patients with hepatitis C]. Gastroenterol Clin Biol. 2000;24(11):1047–51.
162. Nakamura J, Terajima K, Aoyagi Y, Akazawa K. Cost-effectiveness of the national screening program for hepatitis C virus in the general population and the high-risk groups. Tohoku J Exp Med. 2008;215(1):33–42.
163. Singer ME, Younossi ZM. Cost effectiveness of screening for hepatitis C virus in asymptomatic, average-risk adults. Am J Med. 2001;111(8):614–21.
164. Stein K, Dalziel K, Walker A, Jenkins B, Round A, Royle P. Screening for hepatitis C in genito-urinary medicine clinics: a cost utility analysis. J Hepatol. 2003;39(5):814–25.
165. Coffin PO, Scott JD, Golden MR, Sullivan SD. Cost-effectiveness and population outcomes of general population screening for hepatitis C. Clin Infect Dis. 2012;54(9):1259–71.
166. McGarry LJ, Pawar VS, Panchmatia HR, Rubin JL, Davis GL, Younossi ZM et al. Economic model of a birth cohort screening program for hepatitis C virus. Hepatology. 2012;55(5):1344–55.
167. Eckman MH, Talal AH, Gordon SC, Schiff E, Sherman KE. Cost-effectiveness of screening for chronic hepatitis C infection in the United States. Clin Infect Dis. 2013;56(10):1382–93.
168. Liu S, Cipriano LE, Holodniy M, Goldhaber-Fiebert JD. Cost-effectiveness analysis of risk-factor guided and birth-cohort screening for chronic hepatitis C infection in the United States. PLoS One. 2013;8(3):e58975.
169. Lapane KL, Jakiche AF, Sugano D, Weng CS, Carey WD. Hepatitis C infection risk analysis: who should be screened? Comparison of multiple screening strategies based on the National Hepatitis Surveillance Program. Am J Gastroenterol. 1998;93(4):591–6.
170. Wong WW, Tu HA, Feld JJ, Wong T, Krahn M. Cost-effectiveness of screening for hepatitis C in Canada. CMAJ. 2015;187(3):E110–21.
171. Ruggeri M, Coretti S, Gasbarrini A, Cicchetti A. Economic assessment of an anti-HCV screening program in Italy. Value Health. 2013;16(6):965–72.
172. Honeycutt AA, Harris JL, Khavjou O, Buffington J, Jones TS, Rein DB. The costs and impacts of testing for hepatitis C virus antibody in public STD clinics. Public Health Rep. 2007;122 (Suppl 2):55–62.
173. Josset V, Torre JP, Tavolacci MP, Van Rossem-Magnani V, Anselme K, Merle V et al. Efficiency of hepatitis C virus screening strategies in general practice. Gastroenterol Clin Biol. 2004;28(4):351–7.
174. Leal P, Stein K, Rosenberg W. What is the cost utility of screening for hepatitis C virus (HCV) in intravenous drug users? J Med Screen. 1999;6(3):124–31.
175. Stein K, Dalziel K, Walker A, Jenkins B, Round A, Royle P. Screening for hepatitis C in injecting drug users: a cost utility analysis. J Public Health (Oxf). 2004;26(1):61–71.
176. Sutton AJ, Edmunds WJ, Gill ON. Estimating the cost-effectiveness of detecting cases of chronic hepatitis C infection on reception into prison. BMC Public Health. 2006;6:170.
177. Sutton AJ, Edmunds WJ, Sweeting MJ, Gill ON. The cost-effectiveness of screening and treatment for hepatitis C in prisons in England and Wales: a cost-utility analysis. J Viral Hepat. 2008;15(11):797–808.
178. Thompson Coon J, Castelnuovo E, Pitt M, Cramp M, Siebert U, Stein K. Case finding for hepatitis C in primary care: a cost utility analysis. Fam Pract. 2006;23(4):393–406.
179. Tramarin A, Gennaro N, Compostella FA, Gallo C, Wendelaar Bonga LJ, Postma MJ. HCV screening to enable early treatment of hepatitis C: a mathematical model to analyse costs and outcomes in two populations. Curr Pharm Des. 2008;14(17):1655–60.
180. Schackman BR, Leff JA, Barter DM, DiLorenzo MA, Feaster DJ, Metsch LR et al. Cost-effectiveness of rapid hepatitis C virus (HCV) testing and simultaneous rapid HCV and HIV testing in substance abuse treatment programs. Addiction. 2015;110(1):129–43.
181. Cipriano LE, Zaric GS, Holodniy M, Bendavid E, Owens DK, Brandeau ML. Cost effectiveness of screening strategies for early identification of HIV and HCV infection in injection drug users. PLoS One. 2012;7(9):e45176.
182. Jusot JF, Colin C. Cost-effectiveness analysis of strategies for hepatitis C screening in French blood recipients. Eur J Public Health. 2001;11(4):373–9.
183. Linas BP, Wong AY, Schackman BR, Kim AY, Freedberg KA. Cost-effective screening for acute hepatitis C virus infection in HIV-infected men who have sex with men. Clin Infect Dis. 2012;55(2):279–90.
184. Plunkett BA, Grobman WA. Routine hepatitis C virus screening in pregnancy: a cost-effectiveness analysis. Am J Obstet Gynecol. 2005;192(4):1153–61.
185. Urbanus AT, van Keep M, Matser AA, Rozenbaum MH, Weegink CJ, van den Hoek A et al. Is adding HCV screening to the antenatal national screening program in Amsterdam, the Netherlands, cost-effective? PLoS One. 2013;8(8):e70319.
186. Deuffic-Burban S, Abiteboul D, Lot F, Branger M, Bouvet E, Yazdanpanah Y. Costs and cost-effectiveness of different follow-up schedules for detection of occupational hepatitis C virus infection. Gut. 2009;58(1):105–10.
187. Miners AH, Martin NK, Ghosh A, Hickman M, Vickerman P. Assessing the cost-effectiveness of finding cases of hepatitis C infection in UK migrant populations and the value of further research. J Viral Hepat. 2014;21(9):616–23.

188. Martin NK, Hickman M, Miners A, Hutchinson SJ, Taylor A, Vickerman P. Cost-effectiveness of HCV case-finding for people who inject drugs via dried blood spot testing in specialist addiction services and prisons. BMJ Open. 2013;3(8).
189. Martin NK, Vickerman P, Foster GR, Hutchinson SJ, Goldberg DJ, Hickman M. Can antiviral therapy for hepatitis C reduce the prevalence of HCV among injecting drug user populations? A modeling analysis of its prevention utility. J Hepatol. 2011;54(6):1137–44.
190. Brogueira P, Costa A, Miranda A, Peres S, Baptista T, Aldir I et al. Improve screening of HCV infection by targeting high prevalence aged groups: analysis of a cohort of HCV and HIV co-infected patients. J Int AIDS Soc. 2014;17(4 Suppl 3):19601.
191. Kim DD, Hutton DW, Raouf AA, Salama M, Hablas A, Seifeldin IA et al. Cost-effectiveness model for hepatitis C screening and treatment: implications for Egypt and other countries with high prevalence. Glob Public Health. 2015;10(3):296–317.
192. Asrani SK, Davis GL. Impact of birth cohort screening for hepatitis C. Curr Gastroenterol Rep. 2014;16(4):381.
193. Jones L, Bates G, McCoy E, Beynon C, McVeigh J, Bellis M. A systematic review of the effectiveness and cost-effectiveness of interventions aimed at raising awareness and engaging with groups who are at an increased risk of hepatitis B and C infection – final report. Liverpool: Centre for Public Health, Faculty of Health and Applied Social Sciences, Liverpool John Moores University; 2012.
194. Suthar AB, Ford N, Bachanas PJ, Wong VJ, Rajan JS, Saltzman AK et al. Towards universal voluntary HIV testing and counselling: a systematic review and meta-analysis of community-based approaches. PLoS Med. 2013;10(8):e1001496.
195. Sylvestre DL, Loftis JM, Hauser P, Genser S, Cesari H, Borek N et al. Co-occurring hepatitis C, substance use, and psychiatric illness: treatment issues and developing integrated models of care. J Urban Health. 2004;81(4):719–34.
196. Gunn RA, Lee MA, Callahan DB, Gonzales P, Murray PJ, Margolis HS. Integrating hepatitis, STD, and HIV services into a drug rehabilitation program. Am J Prev Med. 2005;29(1):27–33.
197. Mvere D, Constantine NT, Katsawde E, Tobaiwa O, Dambire S, Corcoran P. Rapid and simple hepatitis assays: encouraging results from a blood donor population in Zimbabwe. Bull World Health Organ. 1996;74(1):19–24.
198. Sato K, Ichiyama S, Iinuma Y, Nada T, Shimokata K, Nakashima N. Evaluation of immunochromatographic assay systems for rapid detection of hepatitis B surface antigen and antibody, Dainascreen HBsAg and Dainascreen Ausab. J Clin Microbiol. 1996;34(6):1420–2.
199. Abraham P, Sujatha R, Raghuraman S, Subramaniam T, Sridharan G. Evaluation of two immunochromatographic assays in relation to 'RAPID' screening of HBsAG. Indian J Med Microbiol. 1998;16(1):23–5.
200. Oh J, Kim T, Yoon H, Min H, Lee H, Choi T. Evaluation of Genedia® HBsAg rapid and Genedia® anti-HBs rapid for the screening of HBsAg and anti-HBs. Korean J Clin Pathol. 1999;19(1):114–7.
201. Kaur H, Dhanao J, Oberoi A. Evaluation of rapid kits for detection of HIV, HBsAg and HCV infections. Indian J Med Sci. 2000;54(10):432–4.
202. Lien TX, Tien NT, Chanpong GF, Cuc CT, Yen VT, Soderquist R et al. Evaluation of rapid diagnostic tests for the detection of human immunodeficiency virus types 1 and 2, hepatitis B surface antigen, and syphilis in Ho Chi Minh City, Vietnam. Am J Trop Med Hyg. 2000;62(2):301–9.
203. Raj AA, Subramaniam T, Raghuraman S, Abraham P. Evaluation of an indigenously manufactured rapid immunochromatographic test for detection of HBsAg. Indian J Pathol Microbiol. 2001;44(4):413–4.
204. Clement F, Dewint P, Leroux-Roels G. Evaluation of a new rapid test for the combined detection of hepatitis B virus surface antigen and hepatitis B virus e antigen. J Clin Microbiol. 2002;40(12):4603–6.
205. Lau DT, Ma H, Lemon SM, Doo E, Ghany MG, Miskovsky E et al. A rapid immunochromatographic assay for hepatitis B virus screening. J Viral Hepat. 2003;10(4):331–4.
206. Akanmu AS, Esan OA, Adewuyi JO, Davies AO, Okany CC, Olatunji RO et al. Evaluation of a rapid test kit for detection of HBsAg/eAg in whole blood: a possible method for pre-donation testing. Afr J Med Med Sci. 2006;35(1):5–8.
207. Nyirenda M, Beadsworth MB, Stephany P, Hart CA, Hart IJ, Munthali C et al. Prevalence of infection with hepatitis B and C virus and coinfection with HIV in medical inpatients in Malawi. J Infect. 2008;57(1):72–7.
208. Lin YH, Wang Y, Loua A, Day GJ, Qiu Y, Nadala ECJ et al. Evaluation of a new hepatitis B virus surface antigen rapid test with improved sensitivity. J Clin Microbiol. 2008;46(10):3319–24.
209. Randrianirina F, Carod JF, Ratsima E, Chretien JB, Richard V, Talarmin A. Evaluation of the performance of four rapid tests for detection of hepatitis B surface antigen in Antananarivo, Madagascar. J Virol Methods. 2008;151(2):294–7.
210. Ola SO, Otegbayo JA, Yakubu A, Aje AO, Odaibo GN, Shokunbi W. Pitfalls in diagnosis of hepatitis B virus infection among adult Nigerians. Niger J Clin Pract. 2009;12(4):350–4.
211. Khan J, Lone D, Hameed A, Munim R, Bhatti M, Khattak A et al. Evaluation of the performance of two rapid immunochromatographic tests for detection of hepatitis B surface antigen and anti HCV antibodies using ELISA tested samples. Ann King Edw Med Univ. 2010;16(1):84–7.
212. Davies J, van Oosterhout JJ, Nyirenda M, Bowden J, Moore E, Hart IJ et al. Reliability of rapid testing for hepatitis B in a region of high HIV endemicity. Trans R Soc Trop Med Hyg. 2010;104(2):162–4.

213. Bjoerkvoll B, Viet L, Ol HS, Lan NT, Sothy S, Hoel H et al. Screening test accuracy among potential blood donors of HBsAg, anti-HBc and anti-HCV to detect hepatitis B and C virus infection in rural Cambodia and Vietnam. Southeast Asian J Trop Med Public Health. 2010;41(5):1127–35.

214. Geretti AM, Patel M, Sarfo FS, Chadwick D, Verheyen J, Fraune M et al. Detection of highly prevalent hepatitis B virus coinfection among HIV-seropositive persons in Ghana. J Clin Microbiol. 2010;48(9):3223–30.

215. Hoffmann CJ, Dayal D, Cheyip M, McIntyre JA, Gray GE, Conway S et al. Prevalence and associations with hepatitis B and hepatitis C infection among HIV-infected adults in South Africa. Int J STD AIDS. 2012;23(10):e10–e3.

216. Bottero J, Boyd A, Gozlan J, Lemoine M, Carrat F, Collignon A et al. Performance of rapid tests for detection of HBsAg and anti-HBsAb in a large cohort, France. J Hepatol. 2013;58(3):473–8.

217. Chameera E, Noordeen F, Pandithasundara H, Abeykoon A. Diagnostic efficacy of rapid assays used for the detection of hepatitis B virus surface antigen. Sri Lankan Journal of Infectious Diseases. 2013;3(2):21–7.

218. Franzeck FC, Ngwale R, Msongole B, Hamisi M, Abdul O, Henning L et al. Viral hepatitis and rapid diagnostic test based screening for HBsAg in HIV-infected patients in rural Tanzania. PLoS One. 2013;8(3):e58468.

219. Chevaliez S, Challine D, Naija H, Luu TC, Laperche S, Nadala L et al. Performance of a new rapid test for the detection of hepatitis B surface antigen in various patient populations. J Clin Virol. 2014;59(2):89–93.

220. Erhabor O, Kwaifa I, Bayawa A, Isaac Z, Dorcas I, Sani I. Comparison of ELISA and rapid screening techniques for the detection of HBsAg among blood donors in Usmanu Danfodiyo University Teaching Hospital Sokoto, North Western Nigeria. J Blood Lymph. 2013;4(2):124.

221. Gish RG, Gutierrez JA, Navarro-Cazarez N, Giang K, Adler D, Tran B et al. A simple and inexpensive point-of-care test for hepatitis B surface antigen detection: serological and molecular evaluation. J Viral Hepat. 2014;21(12):905–8.

222. Honge B, Jespersen S, Medina C, Te D, da Silva Z, Ostergaard L et al. Hepatitis B virus surface antigen and anti-hepatitis C virus rapid tests underestimate hepatitis prevalence among HIV-infected patients. HIV Med. 2014;15(9):571–6.

223. Liu C, Chen T, Lin J, Chen H, Chen J, Lin S et al. Evaluation of the performance of four methods for detection of hepatitis B surface antigen and their application for testing 116,455 specimens. J Virol Methods. 2014;196:174–8.

224. Mutocheluh M, Owusu M, Kwofie TB, Akadigo T, Appau E, Narkwa PW. Risk factors associated with hepatitis B exposure and the reliability of five rapid kits commonly used for screening blood donors in Ghana. BMC Res Notes. 2014;7:873.

225. Upreti SR, Gurung S, Patel M, Dixit SM, Krause LK, Shakya G et al. Prevalence of chronic hepatitis B virus infection before and after implementation of a hepatitis B vaccination program among children in Nepal. Vaccine. 2014;32(34):4304–9.

226. Njai HF, Shimakawa Y, Sanneh B, Ferguson L, Ndow G, Mendy M et al. Validation of rapid point-of-care (POC) tests for detection of hepatitis B surface antigen in field and laboratory settings in the Gambia, Western Africa. J Clin Microbiol. 2015;53(4):1156–63.

227. Ol HS, Bjoerkvoll B, Sothy S, Van Heng Y, Hoel H, Husebekk A et al. Prevalence of hepatitis B and hepatitis C virus infections in potential blood donors in rural Cambodia. Southeast Asian J Trop Med Public Health. 2009;40(5):963–71.

228. Peng J, Cheng L, Yin B, Guan Q, Liu Y, Wu S et al. Development of an economic and efficient strategy to detect HBsAg: application of 'gray-zones' in ELISA and combined use of several detection assays. Clin Chim Acta. 2011;412(23–24):2046–51.

229. Viet L, Lan NT, Ty PX, Bjorkvoll B, Hoel H, Gutteberg T et al. Prevalence of hepatitis B & hepatitis C virus infections in potential blood donors in rural Vietnam. Indian J Med Res. 2012;136(1):74–81.

230. Scheiblauer H, El-Nageh M, Diaz S, Nick S, Zeichhardt H, Grunert HP et al. Performance evaluation of 70 hepatitis B virus (HBV) surface antigen (HBsAg) assays from around the world by a geographically diverse panel with an array of HBV genotypes and HBsAg subtypes. Vox Sang. 2010;98(3 Pt 2):403–14.

231. National HBV testing policy. Sydney: Australasian Society for HIV, Viral hepatitis and Sexual Health Medicine; 2012 (http://testingportal.ashm.org.au/images/HepB_TESTING_POLICY_MARCH2014_V1.1_FOR%20PRINT.pdf, accessed 5 February 2017).

232. Gao F, Talbot EA, Loring CH, Power JJ, Dionne-Odom J, Alroy-Preis S et al. Performance of the OraQuick HCV rapid antibody test for screening exposed patients in a hepatitis C outbreak investigation. J Clin Microbiol. 2014;52(7):2650–2.

233. Hess KL, Fisher DG, Reynolds GL. Sensitivity and specificity of point-of-care rapid combination syphilis-HIV-HCV tests. PLoS One. 2014;9(11):e112190.

234. Hui AY, Chan FK, Chan PK, Tam JS, Sung JJ. Evaluation of a new rapid whole-blood serological test for hepatitis c virus. Acta Virol. 2002;46(1):47–8.

235. Lee SR, Kardos KW, Schiff E, Berne CA, Mounzer K, Banks AT et al. Evaluation of a new, rapid test for detecting HCV infection, suitable for use with blood or oral fluid. J Virol Methods. 2011;172(1–2):27–31.

236. Al-Tahish G, El-Barrawy MA, Hashish MH, Heddaya Z. Effectiveness of three types of rapid tests for the detection of hepatitis C virus antibodies among blood donors in Alexandria, Egypt. J Virol Methods. 2013;189(2):370–4.

237. Buti M, Cotrina M, Chan H, Jardi R, Rodriguez F, Costa X et al. Rapid method for the detection of anti-HCV antibodies in patients with chronic hepatitis C. Rev Esp Enferm Dig. 2000;92(3):140–6.
238. Cha YJ, Park Q, Kang ES, Yoo BC, Park KU, Kim JW et al. Performance evaluation of the OraQuick hepatitis C virus rapid antibody test. Ann Lab Med. 2013;33(3):184–9.
239. da Rosa L, Dantas-Correa EB, Narciso-Schiavon JL, Schiavon L de L. Diagnostic performance of two point-of-care tests for anti-HCV detection. Hepat Mon. 2013;13(9):e12274.
240. Ibrahim S, Al Attas SA, Mansour GA, Ouda S, Fallatah H. Accuracy of rapid oral HCV diagnostic test among a Saudi sample. Clin Oral Investig. 2015;19(2):475–80.
241. Jewett A, Smith BD, Garfein RS, Cuevas-Mota J, Teshale EH, Weinbaum CM. Field-based performance of three pre-market rapid hepatitis C virus antibody assays in STAHR (Study to Assess Hepatitis C Risk) among young adults who inject drugs in San Diego, CA. J Clin Virol. 2012;54(3):213–7.
242. Kosack CS, Nick S, Shanks L. Diagnostic accuracy evaluation of the ImmunoFlow HCV rapid immunochromatographic test for the detection of hepatitis C antibodies. J Virol Methods. 2014;204:6–10.
243. Kim MH, Kang SY, Lee WI. Evaluation of a new rapid test kit to detect hepatitis C virus infection. J Virol Methods. 2013;193(2):379–82.
244. Montebugnoli L, Borea G, Miniero R, Sprovieri G. A rapid test for the visual detection of anti-hepatitis C virus antibodies in whole blood. Clin Chim Acta. 1999;288(1–2):91–6.
245. Poovorawan Y, Theamboonlers A, Chumdermpadetsuk S, Thong CP. Comparative results in detection of HCV antibodies by using a rapid HCV test, ELISA and immunoblot. Southeast Asian J Trop Med Public Health. 1994;25(4):647–9.
246. Scalioni Lde P, Cruz HM, de Paula VS, Miguel JC, Marques VA, Villela-Nogueira CA et al. Performance of rapid hepatitis C virus antibody assays among high- and low-risk populations. J Clin Virol. 2014;60(3):200–5.
247. Smith BD, Drobeniuc J, Jewett A, Branson BM, Garfein RS, Teshale E et al. Evaluation of three rapid screening assays for detection of antibodies to hepatitis C virus. J Infect Dis. 2011;204(6):825–31.
248. Yaari A, Tovbin D, Zlotnick M, Mostoslavsky M, Shemer-Avni Y, Hanuka N et al. Detection of HCV salivary antibodies by a simple and rapid test. J Virol Methods. 2006;133(1):1–5.
249. Daniel HD, Abraham P, Raghuraman S, Vivekanandan P, Subramaniam T, Sridharan G. Evaluation of a rapid assay as an alternative to conventional enzyme immunoassays for detection of hepatitis C virus-specific antibodies. J Clin Microbiol. 2005;43(4):1977–8.
250. Drobnik A, Judd C, Banach D, Egger J, Konty K, Rude E. Public health implications of rapid hepatitis C screening with an oral swab for community-based organizations serving high-risk populations. Am J Public Health. 2011;101(11):2151–5.
251. Lee SR, Yearwood GD, Guillon GB, Kurtz LA, Fischl M, Friel T et al. Evaluation of a rapid, point-of-care test device for the diagnosis of hepatitis C infection. J Clin Virol. 2010;48(1):15–7.
252. Njouom R, Tejiokem MC, Zanga MC, Pouillot R, Ayouba A, Pasquier C et al. A cost-effective algorithm for the diagnosis of hepatitis C virus infection and prediction of HCV viremia in Cameroon. J Virol Methods. 2006;133(2):223–6.
253. O'Connell RJ, Gates RG, Bautista CT, Imbach M, Eggleston JC, Beardsley SG et al. Laboratory evaluation of rapid test kits to detect hepatitis C antibody for use in predonation screening in emergency settings. Transfusion. 2013;53(3):505–17.
254. Yuen MF, Hui CK, Yuen JC, Young JL, Lai CL. The accuracy of SM-HCV rapid test for the detection of antibody to hepatitis C virus. Am J Gastroenterol. 2001;96(3):838–41.
255. Lee S, Kardos K, Yearwood G, Kurtz L, Roehler M, Feiss G. Results of a multi-center evaluation of a new rapid test for detection of HCV infection using whole blood, serum, plasma and oral fluid. J Hepatol. 2010;52(Suppl. 1):S271.
256. Larrat S, Bourdon C, Baccard M, Garnaud C, Mathieu S, Quesada JL et al. Performance of an antigen-antibody combined assay for hepatitis C virus testing without venipuncture. J Clin Virol. 2012;55(3):220–5.
257. Smith BD, Teshale E, Jewett A, Weinbaum CM, Neaigus A, Hagan H et al. Performance of premarket rapid hepatitis C virus antibody assays in 4 national human immunodeficiency virus behavioral surveillance system sites. Clin Infect Dis. 2011;53(8):780–6.
258. Mullis CE, Laeyendecker O, Reynolds SJ, Ocama P, Quinn J, Boaz I et al. High frequency of false-positive hepatitis C virus enzyme-linked immunosorbent assay in Rakai, Uganda. Clin Infect Dis. 2013;57(12):1747–50.
259. Barreto AM, Takei K, E CS, Bellesa MA, Salles NA, Barreto CC et al. Cost-effective analysis of different algorithms for the diagnosis of hepatitis C virus infection. Braz J Med Biol Res. 2008;41(2):126–34.
260. Bonacini M, Lin HJ, Hollinger FB. Effect of coexisting HIV-1 infection on the diagnosis and evaluation of hepatitis C virus. J Acquir Immune Defic Syndr. 2001;26(4):340–4.
261. George SL, Gebhardt J, Klinzman D, Foster MB, Patrick KD, Schmidt WN et al. Hepatitis C virus viremia in HIV-infected individuals with negative HCV antibody tests. J Acquir Immune Defic Syndr. 2002;31(2):154–62.
262. Thio CL, Nolt KR, Astemborski J, Vlahov D, Nelson KE, Thomas DL. Screening for hepatitis C virus in human immunodeficiency virus-infected individuals. J Clin Microbiol. 2000;38(2):575–7.

263. Thomson EC, Nastouli E, Main J, Karayiannis P, Eliahoo J, Muir D et al. Delayed anti-HCV antibody response in HIV-positive men acutely infected with HCV. AIDS. 2009;23(1):89–93.
264. Lok AS, McMahon BJ. Chronic hepatitis B: update 2009. Hepatology. 2009;50(3):661–2.
265. Brunetto MR, Oliveri F, Colombatto P, Moriconi F, Ciccorossi P, Coco B et al. Hepatitis B surface antigen serum levels help to distinguish active from inactive hepatitis B virus genotype D carriers. Gastroenterology. 2010;139(2):483–90.
266. Chen CJ, Iloeje UH, Yang HI. Long-term outcomes in hepatitis B: the REVEAL-HBV study. Clin Liver Dis. 2007;11(4):797–816.
267. Gerlach JT, Diepolder HM, Zachoval R, Gruener NH, Jung MC, Ulsenheimer A et al. Acute hepatitis C: high rate of both spontaneous and treatment-induced viral clearance. Gastroenterology. 2003;125(1):80–8.
268. UNITAID. Hepatitis C diagnostic technology landscape. Geneva: World Health Organization; 2015 (http://unitaid.org/images/marketdynamics/publications/UNITAID-HCV_Diagnostic_Landscape-1st_edition.pdf, accessed 5 February 2017).
269. Tanaka E, Kiyosawa K, Matsumoto A, Kashiwakuma T, Hasegawa A, Mori H et al. Serum levels of hepatitis C virus core protein in patients with chronic hepatitis C treated with interferon alfa. Hepatology. 1996;23(6):1330–3.
270. Tillmann HL. Hepatitis C virus core antigen testing: role in diagnosis, disease monitoring and treatment. World J Gastroenterol. 2014;20(22):6701–6.
271. Freiman JM, Tran TM, Schumacher SG, White LF, Ongarello S, Cohn J et al. Hepatitis C core antigen testing for diagnosis of hepatitis C virus infection: a systematic review and meta-analysis. Ann Intern Med. 2016;165(5):345–55.
272. Lee SC, Antony A, Lee N, Leibow J, Yang JQ, Soviero S et al. Improved version 2.0 qualitative and quantitative AMPLICOR reverse transcription-PCR tests for hepatitis C virus RNA: calibration to international units, enhanced genotype reactivity, and performance characteristics. J Clin Microbiol. 2000;38(11):4171–9.
273. Yu ML, Chuang WL, Dai CY, Chen SC, Lin ZY, Hsieh MY et al. Clinical evaluation of the automated COBAS AMPLICOR HCV MONITOR test version 2.0 for quantifying serum hepatitis C virus RNA and comparison to the quantiplex HCV version 2.0 test. J Clin Microbiol. 2000;38(8):2933–9.
274. Sabato MF, Shiffman ML, Langley MR, Wilkinson DS, Ferreira-Gonzalez A. Comparison of performance characteristics of three real-time reverse transcription-PCR test systems for detection and quantification of hepatitis C virus. J Clin Microbiol. 2007;45(8):2529–36.
275. Vermehren J, Kau A, Gartner BC, Gobel R, Zeuzem S, Sarrazin C. Differences between two real-time PCR-based hepatitis C virus (HCV) assays (RealTime HCV and Cobas AmpliPrep/Cobas TaqMan) and one signal amplification assay (Versant HCV RNA 3.0) for RNA detection and quantification. J Clin Microbiol. 2008;46(12):3880–91.
276. Vermehren J, Susser S, Berger A, Perner D, Peiffer KH, Allwinn R et al. Clinical utility of the ARCHITECT HCV Ag assay for early treatment monitoring in patients with chronic hepatitis C genotype 1 infection. J Clin Virol. 2012;55(1):17–22.
277. European Association for the Study of the Liver. EASL Clinical Practice Guidelines: management of hepatitis C virus infection. J Hepatol. 2014;60(2):392–420. (http://www.easl.eu/medias/cpg/HEPC-revised-version/English-report.pdf, accessed 5 February 2017).
278. Ghany MG, Nelson DR, Strader DB, Thomas DL, Seeff LB. An update on treatment of genotype 1 chronic hepatitis C virus infection: 2011 practice guideline by the American Association for the Study of Liver Diseases. Hepatology. 2011;54(4):1433–44.
279. Loggi E, Cursaro C, Scuteri A, Grandini E, Panno AM, Galli S et al. Patterns of HCV-RNA and HCV core antigen in the early monitoring of standard treatment for chronic hepatitis C. J Clin Virol. 2013;56(3):207–11.
280. Fujino T, Nakamuta M, Aoyagi Y, Fukuizumi K, Takemoto R, Yoshimoto T et al. Early decline of the HCV core antigen can predict SVR in patients with HCV treated by pegylated interferon plus ribavirin combination therapy. J Dig Dis. 2009;10(1):21–5.
281. Takahashi M, Saito H, Higashimoto M, Atsukawa K, Ishii H. Benefit of hepatitis C virus core antigen assay in prediction of therapeutic response to interferon and ribavirin combination therapy. J Clin Microbiol. 2005;43(1):186–91.
282. Feng B, Yang RF, Xie Q, Shang J, Kong FY, Zhang HY et al. Hepatitis C virus core antigen, an earlier and stronger predictor on sustained virological response in patients with genotype 1 HCV infection. BMC Gastroenterol. 2014;14:47.
283. Moscato GA, Giannelli G, Grandi B, Pieri D, Marsi O, Guarducci I et al. Quantitative determination of hepatitis C core antigen in therapy monitoring for chronic hepatitis C. Intervirology. 2011;54(2):61–5.
284. Gu J, Yu T, Liang Z. Performances of HCV Ag or HCV RNA kits for screening of HCV-infected samples. Chinese Journal of Biologicals. 2014;27(9):1181–4.
285. van Helden J, Weiskirchen R. Hepatitis C diagnostics: clinical evaluation of the HCV-core antigen determination. Z Gastroenterol. 2014;52(10):1164–70.
286. Schnuriger A, Dominguez S, Valantin MA, Tubiana R, Duvivier C, Ghosn J et al. Early detection of hepatitis C virus infection using a new combined antigen-antibody detection assay: potential use in HIV co-infected individuals. Pathol Biol (Paris). 2007;54(10):578–86.

287. Okazaki K, Nishiyama Y, Saitou T, Shibata N, Yamamoto C, Oosaga J et al. Fundamental evaluation of HCV core antigen method comparison with Cobas Amplicor HCV monitor v2.0 (high range method). Rinsho Byori. 2008;56(2):95–100.
288. Sidharthan S, Kohli A, Sims Z, Nelson A, Osinusi A, Masur H et al. Utility of hepatitis C viral load monitoring on direct-acting antiviral therapy. Clin Infect Dis. 2015;60(12):1743–51.
289. Snijdewind IJ, van Kampen JJ, Fraaij PL, van der Ende ME, Osterhaus AD, Gruters RA. Current and future applications of dried blood spots in viral disease management. Antiviral Res. 2012;93(3):309–21.
290. Grüner N, Stambouli O, Ross RS. Dried blood spots – preparing and processing for use in immunoassays and in molecular techniques. J Vis Exp. 2015(97):52619.
291. McDade TW, Williams S, Snodgrass JJ. What a drop can do: dried blood spots as a minimally invasive method for integrating biomarkers into population-based research. Demography. 2007;44(4):899–925.
292. Hirtz C, Lehmann S. Blood sampling using "dried blood spot": a clinical biology revolution underway? Ann Biol Clin (Paris). 2015;73(1):25–37.
293. Ross RS, Stambouli O, Gruner N, Marcus U, Cai W, Zhang W et al. Detection of infections with hepatitis B virus, hepatitis C virus, and human immunodeficiency virus by analyses of dried blood spots – performance characteristics of the ARCHITECT system and two commercial assays for nucleic acid amplification. Virol J. 2013;10:72.
294. Greenman J, Roberts T, Cohn J, Messac L. Dried blood spot in the genotyping, quantification and storage of HCV RNA: a systematic literature review. J Viral Hepat. 2015;22(4):353–61.
295. Jones L, Bates G, McCoy E, Beynon C, McVeigh J, Bellis MA. Effectiveness of interventions to increase hepatitis C testing uptake among high-risk groups: a systematic review. Eur J Public Health. 2014;24(5):781–8.
296. Boa-Sorte N, Purificacao A, Amorim T, Assuncao L, Reis A, Galvao-Castro B. Dried blood spot testing for the antenatal screening of HTLV, HIV, syphilis, toxoplasmosis and hepatitis B and C: prevalence, accuracy and operational aspects. Braz J Infect Dis. 2014;18(6):618–24.
297. Forbi JC, Obagu JO, Gyar SD, Pam CR, Pennap GR, Agwale SM. Application of dried blood spot in the sero-diagnosis of hepatitis B infection (HBV) in an HBV hyper-endemic nation. Ann Afr Med. 2010;9(1):44–5.
298. Kania D, Bekale AM, Nagot N, Mondain AM, Ottomani L, Meda N et al. Combining rapid diagnostic tests and dried blood spot assays for point-of-care testing of human immunodeficiency virus, hepatitis B and hepatitis C infections in Burkina Faso, West Africa. Clin Microbiol Infect. 2013;19(12):E533–41.
299. Lee CE, Sri Ponnampalavanar S, Syed Omar SF, Mahadeva S, Ong LY, Kamarulzaman A. Evaluation of the dried blood spot (DBS) collection method as a tool for detection of HIV Ag/Ab, HBsAg, anti-HBs and anti-HCV in a Malaysian tertiary referral hospital. Ann Acad Med Singapore. 2011;40(10):448–53.
300. Mendy M, Kirk GD, van der Sande M, Jeng-Barry A, Lesi OA, Hainaut P et al. Hepatitis B surface antigenaemia and alpha-foetoprotein detection from dried blood spots: applications to field-based studies and to clinical care in hepatitis B virus endemic areas. J Viral Hepat. 2005;12(6):642–7.
301. Mohamed S, Raimondo A, Penaranda G, Camus C, Ouzan D, Ravet S et al. Dried blood spot sampling for hepatitis B virus serology and molecular testing. PLoS One. 2013;8(4):e61077.
302. Villa E, Cartolari R, Bellentani S, Rivasi P, Casolo G, Manenti F. Hepatitis B virus markers on dried blood spots. A new tool for epidemiological research. J Clin Pathol. 1981;34(7):809–12.
303. Villar LM, de Oliveira JC, Cruz HM, Yoshida CF, Lampe E, Lewis-Ximenez LL. Assessment of dried blood spot samples as a simple method for detection of hepatitis B virus markers. J Med Virol. 2011;83(9):1522–9.
304. Brandao CP, Marques BL, Marques VA, Villela-Nogueira CA, Do OK, de Paula MT et al. Simultaneous detection of hepatitis C virus antigen and antibodies in dried blood spots. J Clin Virol. 2013;57(2):98–102.
305. Tuaillon E, Mondain AM, Meroueh F, Ottomani L, Picot MC, Nagot N et al. Dried blood spot for hepatitis C virus serology and molecular testing. Hepatology. 2010;51(3):752–8.
306. O'Brien J, Kruzel K, Wandell M, Vinogradov I, Sheagren J, Frank A. Detection of hepatitis C antibody with at-home collection kits using an innovative laboratory algorithm. Infect Disin Clin Pract. 2001;10(9):474–80.
307. Croom HA, Richards KM, Best SJ, Francis BH, Johnson EI, Dax EM et al. Commercial enzyme immunoassay adapted for the detection of antibodies to hepatitis C virus in dried blood spots. J Clin Virol. 2006;36(1):68–71.
308. Marques BL, Brandao CU, Silva EF, Marques VA, Villela-Nogueira CA, Do OK et al. Dried blood spot samples: optimization of commercial EIAs for hepatitis C antibody detection and stability under different storage conditions. J Med Virol. 2012;84(10):1600–7.
309. Waterboer T, Dondog B, Michael KM, Michel A, Schmitt M, Vaccarella S et al. Dried blood spot samples for seroepidemiology of infections with human papillomaviruses, Helicobacter pylori, hepatitis C virus, and JC virus. Cancer Epidemiol Biomarkers Prev. 2012;21(2):287–93.
310. Nandagopal P, Iqbal HS, Saravanan S, Solomon SS, Mehta S, Selvakumar M et al. Evaluation of dried blood spot as an alternative specimen for the diagnosis of anti-HCV in resource-limited settings. Indian J Med Microbiol. 2014;32(2):208–10.
311. Dokubo EK, Evans J, Winkelman V, Cyrus S, Tobler LH, Asher A et al. Comparison of hepatitis C virus RNA and antibody detection in dried blood spots and plasma specimens. J Clin Virol. 2014;59(4):223–7.

312. Tejada-Strop A, Drobeniuc J, Mixson-Hayden T, Forbi JC, Le NT, Li L et al. Disparate detection outcomes for anti-HCV IgG and HCV RNA in dried blood spots. J Virol Methods. 2015;212:66–70.
313. Chevaliez S, Soulier A, Poiteau L, Pawlotsky JM. Dried blood spots (DBS), a promising tool for large-scale hepatitis C screening, diagnosis and treatment monitoring. International Liver Congress 2014. 49th Annual Meeting of the European Association for the Study of the Liver (EASL), 9–13 April 2014, London. J Hepatol. 2014;60 (1 Suppl):S325–S326. [Abstract P765]
314. Parker SP, Cubitt WD, Ades AE. A method for the detection and confirmation of antibodies to hepatitis C virus in dried blood spots. J Virol Methods. 1997;68(2):199–205.
315. Lukacs Z, Dietrich A, Ganschow R, Kohlschutter A, Kruithof R. Simultaneous determination of HIV antibodies, hepatitis C antibodies, and hepatitis B antigens in dried blood spots – a feasibility study using a multi-analyte immunoassay. Clin Chem Lab Med. 2005;43(2):141–5.
316. McCarron B, Fox R, Wilson K, Cameron S, McMenamin J, McGregor G et al. Hepatitis C antibody detection in dried blood spots. J Viral Hepat. 1999;6(6):453–6.
317. Shepherd SJ, Kean J, Hutchinson SJ, Cameron SO, Goldberg DJ, Carman WF et al. A hepatitis C avidity test for determining recent and past infections in both plasma and dried blood spots. J Clin Virol. 2013;57(1):29–35.
318. Alidjinou EK, Moukassa D, Sane F, Twagirimana Nyenyeli S, Akoko EC, Mountou MV et al. Detection of hepatitis B virus infection markers in dried plasma spots among patients in Congo-Brazzaville. Diagn Microbiol Infect Dis. 2014;78(3):229–31.
319. Alhusseini N, Abadeer M, El-Taher S. Hepatitis B virus DNA can be amplified directly from dried blood spot on filter paper. Am J Biochem Biotechnol. 2012;8(2):143–9.
320. Durgadevi S, Dhodapkar R, Parija S. Serological and molecular diagnosis of hepatitis B virus. BMC Infect Dis. 2012;12(Suppl 1):P31.
321. Gupta BP, Jayasuryan N, Jameel S. Direct detection of hepatitis B virus from dried blood spots by polymerase chain reaction amplification. J Clin Microbiol. 1992;30(8):1913–6.
322. Halfon P, Raimondo A, Ouzan D, Bourlière M, Khiri H, Cohen-Bacrie S et al. Dried blood spot for hepatitis B virus serology and molecular testing. International Liver Congress 2012. 47th Annual Meeting of the European Association for the Study of the Liver (EASL), 18–22 April 2012. Barcelona. J Hepatol. 2012;56 (Suppl 2):S62. [Abstract 142]
323. Jardi R, Rodriguez-Frias F, Buti M, Schaper M, Valdes A, Martinez M et al. Usefulness of dried blood samples for quantification and molecular characterization of HBV-DNA. Hepatology. 2004;40(1):133–9.
324. Lira R, Maldonado-Rodriguez A, Rojas-Montes O, Ruiz-Tachiquin M, Torres-Ibarra R, Cano-Dominguez C et al. Use of dried blood samples for monitoring hepatitis B virus infection. Virol J. 2009;6:153.
325. Vinikoor MJ, Zurcher S, Musukuma K, Kachuwaire O, Rauch A, Chi BH et al. Hepatitis B viral load in dried blood spots: a validation study in Zambia. J Clin Virol. 2015;72:20–4.
326. Abe K, Konomi N. Hepatitis C virus RNA in dried serum spotted onto filter paper is stable at room temperature. J Clin Microbiol. 1998;36(10):3070–2.
327. Bennett S, Gunson RN, McAllister GE, Hutchinson SJ, Goldberg DJ, Cameron SO et al. Detection of hepatitis C virus RNA in dried blood spots. J Clin Virol. 2012;54(2):106–9.
328. De Crignis E, Re MC, Cimatti L, Zecchi L, Gibellini D. HIV-1 and HCV detection in dried blood spots by SYBR Green multiplex real-time RT-PCR. J Virol Methods. 2010;165(1):51–6.
329. Soulier A, Poiteau L, Rosa I, Hezode C, Roudot-Thoraval F, Pawlotsky JM et al. Dried blood spots: a tool to ensure broad access to hepatitis C screening, diagnosis, and treatment monitoring. J Infect Dis. 2016;213(7):1087–95.
330. Santos C, Reis A, Dos Santos CV, Damas C, Silva MH, Viana MV et al. The use of real-time PCR to detect hepatitis C virus RNA in dried blood spots from Brazilian patients infected chronically. J Virol Methods. 2012;179(1):17–20.
331. Solmone M, Girardi E, Costa F, Pucillo L, Ippolito G, Capobianchi MR. Simple and reliable method for detection and genotyping of hepatitis C virus RNA in dried blood spots stored at room temperature. J Clin Microbiol. 2002;40(9):3512–4.
332. Solmone M, Girardi E, Costa F, Ippolito G, Capobianchi MR. Simple and reliable method for HCV-RNA detection/genotyping in dried blood spots. J Hepatol. 2002;36(Suppl 1):131.
333. Craine N, Whitaker R, Perrett S, Zou L, Hickman M, Lyons M. A stepped wedge cluster randomized control trial of dried blood spot testing to improve the uptake of hepatitis C antibody testing within UK prisons. Eur J Public Health. 2015;25(2):351–7.
334. Hickman M, McDonald T, Judd A, Nichols T, Hope V, Skidmore S et al. Increasing the uptake of hepatitis C virus testing among injecting drug users in specialist drug treatment and prison settings by using dried blood spots for diagnostic testing: a cluster randomized controlled trial. J Viral Hepat. 2008;15(4):250–4.
335. Hutchinson SJ, Dillon JF, Fox R, McDonald SA, Innes HA, Weir A et al. Expansion of HCV treatment access to people who have injected drugs through effective translation of research into public health policy: Scotland's experience. Int J Drug Policy. 2015;26(11):1041–9.
336. Hepatitis B and C: ways to promote and offer testing to people at increased risk of infection. London: National Institute for Health and Clinical Excellence (NICE); 2012 (https:// https://www.nice.org.uk/guidance/ph43/resources/hepatitis-b-and-c-ways-to-promote-and-offer-testing-draft-guidance2, accessed 6 February 2017).

337. McLeod A, Weir A, Aitken C, Gunson R, Templeton K, Molyneaux P et al. Rise in testing and diagnosis associated with Scotland's Action Plan on Hepatitis C and introduction of dried blood spot testing. J Epidemiol Community Health. 2014;68(12):1182–8.

338. Place des tests rapides d'orientation diagnostique (TROD) dans la stratégie de dépistage de l'hépatite C. Saint-Denis La Plaine Cedex: Haute Autorité Sanitaire; 2014 (http://www.has-sante.fr/portail/upload/docs/application/pdf/2014-05/place_des_trod_dans_la_strategie_de_depistage_de_vhc-_rapport.pdf, accessed 6 February 2017).

339. Bravo MJ, Vallejo F, Barrio G, Brugal MT, Molist G, Pulido J et al. HCV seroconversion among never-injecting heroin users at baseline: no predictors identified other than starting injection. Int J Drug Policy. 2012;23(5):415–9.

340. Allen EJ, Palmateer NE, Hutchinson SJ, Cameron S, Goldberg DJ, Taylor A. Association between harm reduction intervention uptake and recent hepatitis C infection among people who inject drugs attending sites that provide sterile injecting equipment in Scotland. Int J Drug Policy. 2012;23(5):346–52.

341. Allard NL, MacLachlan JH, Cowie BC. The cascade of care for Australians living with chronic hepatitis B: measuring access to diagnosis, management and treatment. Aust N Z J Public Health. 2015;39(3):255–9.

342. Yehia BR, Schranz AJ, Umscheid CA, Lo Re V 3rd. The treatment cascade for chronic hepatitis C virus infection in the United States: a systematic review and meta-analysis. PLoS One. 2014;9(7):e101554.

343. Govindasamy D, Ford N, Kranzer K. Risk factors, barriers and facilitators for linkage to antiretroviral therapy care: a systematic review. AIDS. 2012;26(16):2059–67.

344. Willenbring ML. Integrating care for patients with infectious, psychiatric, and substance use disorders: concepts and approaches. AIDS. 2005;19 Suppl 3:S227–37.

345. Ahmed I, Habibi B, Iqbal J, Niaz Z, Naqvi A. Improving outcome in hepatitis C management: a need for dedicated multi-disciplinary service to improve compliance with treatment. J Gastroenterol Hepatol Res. 2013;2(8):737–9.

346. Arora S, Thornton K, Murata G, Deming P, Kalishman S, Dion D et al. Outcomes of treatment for hepatitis C virus infection by primary care providers. N Engl J Med. 2011;364(23):2199–207.

347. Asthana A, Choong J, Lubel J. Education does not improve hepatitis B screening uptake in those receiving cytotoxic chemotherapy – time for alternative strategies. J Gastroenterol Hepatol. 2012;27:162.

348. Bastani R, Glenn BA, Maxwell AE, Jo AM, Herrmann AK, Crespi CM et al. Cluster-randomized trial to increase hepatitis B testing among Koreans in Los Angeles. Cancer Epidemiol Biomarkers Prev. 2015;24(9):1341–9.

349. Bonkovsky HL, Tice AD, Yapp RG, Bodenheimer HC Jr, Monto A, Rossi SJ et al. Efficacy and safety of peginterferon alfa-2a/ribavirin in methadone maintenance patients: randomized comparison of direct observed therapy and self-administration. Am J Gastroenterol. 2008;103(11):2757–65.

350. Bruce RD, Eiserman J, Acosta A, Gote C, Lim JK, Altice FL. Developing a modified directly observed therapy intervention for hepatitis C treatment in a methadone maintenance program: implications for program replication. Am J Drug Alcohol Abuse. 2012;38(3):206–12.

351. Cacoub P, Ouzan D, Melin P, Lang JP, Rotily M, Fontanges T et al. Patient education improves adherence to peg-interferon and ribavirin in chronic genotype 2 or 3 hepatitis C virus infection: a prospective, real-life, observational study. World J Gastroenterol. 2008;14(40):6195–203.

352. Carrion JA, Gonzalez-Colominas E, Garcia-Retortillo M, Canete N, Cirera I, Coll S et al. A multidisciplinary support programme increases the efficiency of pegylated interferon alfa-2a and ribavirin in hepatitis C. J Hepatol. 2013;59(5):926–33.

353. Chakrabarty G, Rice P, Forton D. Randomized controlled trial of home-based self-administered dried blood spot testing versus written advice for community screening of hepatitis B contacts. Hepatology. 2013;58:616A.

354. Chen MS Jr, Fang DM, Stewart SL, Ly MY, Lee S, Dang JH et al. Increasing hepatitis B screening for hmong adults: results from a randomized controlled community-based study. Cancer Epidemiol Biomarkers Prev. 2013;22(5):782–91.

355. Chen JY, Feeney ER, Chung RT. HCV and HIV co-infection: mechanisms and management. Nat Rev Gastroenterol Hepatol. 2014;11(6):362–71.

356. Cioe PA, Stein MD, Promrat K, Friedmann PD. A comparison of modified directly observed therapy to standard care for chronic hepatitis C. J Community Health. 2013;38(4):679–84.

357. Craine N, Parry J, O'Toole J, D'Arcy S, Lyons M. Improving blood-borne viral diagnosis; clinical audit of the uptake of dried blood spot testing offered by a substance misuse service. J Viral Hepat. 2009;16(3):219–22.

358. Cullen W, Stanley J, Langton D, Kelly Y, Staines A, Bury G. Hepatitis C infection among injecting drug users in general practice: a cluster randomised controlled trial of clinical guidelines' implementation. Br J Gen Pract. 2006;56(532):848–56.

359. Curcio F, Di Martino F, Capraro C, Angelucci F, Bulla F, Caprio N et al. Together ... to take care: multidisciplinary management of hepatitis C virus treatment in randomly selected drug users with chronic hepatitis. J Addict Med. 2010;4(4):223–32.

360. Drainoni ML, Litwin AH, Smith BD, Koppelman EA, McKee MD, Christiansen CL et al. Effectiveness of a risk screener in identifying hepatitis C virus in a primary care setting. Am J Public Health. 2012;102(11):e115–21.

361. Evon DM, Simpson K, Kixmiller S, Galanko J, Dougherty K, Golin C et al. A randomized controlled trial of an integrated care intervention to increase eligibility for chronic hepatitis C treatment. Am J Gastroenterol. 2011;106(10):1777–86.

362. Hagedorn H, Dieperink E, Dingmann D, Durfee J, Ho SB, Isenhart C et al. Integrating hepatitis prevention services into a substance use disorder clinic. J Subst Abuse Treat. 2007;32(4):391–8.

363. Helsper CW, van Essen GA, Bonten MJ, de Wit NJ. A support programme for primary care leads to substantial improvements in the effectiveness of a public hepatitis C campaign. Fam Pract. 2010;27(3):328–32.

364. Hirsch AA, Lawrence RH, Kern E, Falck-Ytter Y, Shumaker DT, Watts B. Implementation and evaluation of a multicomponent quality improvement intervention to improve efficiency of hepatitis C screening and diagnosis. Jt Comm J Qual Patient Saf. 2014;40(8):351–7.

365. Ho SB, Brau N, Cheung R, Liu L, Sanchez C, Sklar M et al. Integrated care increases treatment and improves outcomes of patients with chronic hepatitis C virus infection and psychiatric illness or substance abuse. Clin Gastroenterol Hepatol. 2015;13(11):2005–14.e3

366. Hsu L, Bowlus CL, Stewart SL, Nguyen TT, Dang J, Chan B et al. Electronic messages increase hepatitis B screening in at-risk Asian American patients: a randomized, controlled trial. Dig Dis Sci. 2013;58(3):807 14.

367. Hussein M, Benner JS, Lee D, Sesti AM, Battleman DS, Brock-Wood C. Propensity score matching in the evaluation of drug therapy management programs: an illustrative analysis of a program for patients with hepatitis C virus. Qual Manag Health Care. 2010;19(1):25–33.

368. Juon HS, Lee S, Strong C, Rimal R, Kirk GD, Bowie J. Effect of a liver cancer education program on hepatitis B screening among Asian Americans in the Baltimore-Washington metropolitan area, 2009–2010. Prev Chronic Dis. 2014;11:130258.

369. Knott A, Dieperink E, Willenbring ML, Heit S, Durfee JM, Wingert M et al. Integrated psychiatric/medical care in a chronic hepatitis C clinic: effect on antiviral treatment evaluation and outcomes. Am J Gastroenterol. 2006;101(10):2254–62.

370. Koruk I, Koruk S, Çopur AC, Simsek Z. A intervention study to improve HBsAg testing and preventive practices for hepatitis B in an obstetrics hospital. TAF Prev Med Bull. 2011;10(3):287–92.

371. Krauskopf K, Kil N, Sofianou A, Toribio W, Lyons J, Singer M et al. Evaluation of an electronic health record prompt for hepatitis c antibody screening of baby boomers in primary care – a cluster randomized control trial. J Gen Intern Med. 2014;29:S88–S9.

372. Larrey D, Salse A, Ribard D, Boutet O, Hyrailles-Blanc V, Niang B et al. Education by a nurse increases response of patients with chronic hepatitis C to therapy with peginterferon-alpha2a and ribavirin. Clin Gastroenterol Hepatol. 2011;9(9):781–5.

373. Lee R, Vu K, Bell CM, Hicks LK. Screening for hepatitis B surface antigen before chemotherapy: current practice and opportunities for improvement. Curr Oncol. 2010;17(6):32–8.

374. Litwin AH, Smith BD, Drainoni ML, McKee D, Gifford AL, Koppelman E et al. Primary care-based interventions are associated with increases in hepatitis C virus testing for patients at risk. Dig Liver Dis. 2012;44(6):497–503.

375. Lubega S, Agbim U, Surjadi M, Mahoney M, Khalili M. Formal hepatitis C education enhances HCV care coordination, expedites HCV treatment and improves antiviral response. Liver Int. 2013;33(7):999–1007.

376. Ma GX, Gao W, Tan Y, Chae WG, Rhee J. A community-based participatory approach to a hepatitis B intervention for Korean Americans. Prog Community Health Partnersh. 2012;6(1):7–16.

377. Masson CL, Delucchi KL, McKnight C, Hettema J, Khalili M, Min A et al. A randomized trial of a hepatitis care coordination model in methadone maintenance treatment. Am J Public Health. 2013;103(10):e81–e8.

378. Matthews H, McLeod M, Oakes K, McCurdy G, Zuckerman M, Carey I et al. Perinatal hepatitis B in a high prevalence inner city population: direct electronic referral improves care. Gut. 2012;61:A79–A80.

379. Merchant RC, Baird JR, Liu T, Taylor LE, Montague BT, Nirenberg TD. Brief intervention to increase emergency department uptake of combined rapid human immunodeficiency virus and hepatitis C screening among a drug misusing population. Acad Emerg Med. 2014;21(7):752–67.

380. Mostert MC, Richardus JH, de Man RA. Referral of chronic hepatitis B patients from primary to specialist care: making a simple guideline work. J Hepatol. 2004;41(6):1026–30.

381. Neri S, Bertino G, Petralia A, Giancarlo C, Rizzotto A, Calvagno GS et al. A multidisciplinary therapeutic approach for reducing the risk of psychiatric side effects in patients with chronic hepatitis C treated with pegylated interferon alpha and ribavirin. J Clin Gastroenterol. 2010;44(9):e210–7.

382. Ramsey SE, Engler PA, Stein MD, Brown RA, Cioe P, Kahler CW et al. Effect of CBT on depressive symptoms in methadone maintenance patients undergoing treatment for hepatitis C. J Addict Res Ther. 2011;2(2):2–10.

383. Reimer J, Schmidt CS, Schulte B, Gansefort D, Golz J, Gerken G et al. Psychoeducation improves hepatitis C virus treatment during opioid substitution therapy: a controlled, prospective multicenter trial. Clin Infect Dis. 2013;57 (Suppl 2):S97–104.

384. Rifai MA, Moles JK, Lehman LP, Van der Linden BJ. Hepatitis C screening and treatment outcomes in patients with substance use/dependence disorders. Psychosomatics. 2006;47(2):112–21.

385. Rosenberg SD, Goldberg RW, Dixon LB, Wolford GL, Slade EP, Himelhoch S et al. Assessing the STIRR model of best practices for blood-borne infections of clients with severe mental illness. Psychiatr Serv. 2010;61(9):885–91.

386. Sahajian F, Excler G, Bailly F, Caillat-Vallet E, Trepo C, Sepetjan M et al. Hepatitis C screening practices among private practitioners: impact of an information campaign. Gastroenterol Clin Biol. 2004;28(8–9):714–9.

387. Tait JM, McIntyre PG, McLeod S, Nathwani D, Dillon JF. The impact of a managed care network on attendance, follow-up and treatment at a hepatitis C specialist centre. J Viral Hepat. 2010;17(10):698–704.

388. Taylor VM, Bastani R, Burke N, Talbot J, Sos C, Liu Q et al. Evaluation of a hepatitis B lay health worker intervention for Cambodian Americans. J Community Health. 2013;38(3):546–53.

389. Taylor VM, Gregory Hislop T, Bajdik C, Teh C, Lam W, Acorda E et al. Hepatitis B ESL education for Asian immigrants. J Community Health. 2011;36(1):35–41.

390. Taylor VM, Hislop TG, Tu SP, Teh C, Acorda E, Yip MP et al. Evaluation of a hepatitis B lay health worker intervention for Chinese Americans and Canadians. J Community Health. 2009;34(3):165–72.

391. van der Veen YJ, van Empelen P, de Zwart O, Visser H, Mackenbach JP, Richardus JH. Cultural tailoring to promote hepatitis B screening in Turkish Dutch: a randomized control study. Health Promot Int. 2014;29(4):692–704.

392. Le Lan C, Guillygomarc'h A, Danielou H, Le Dreau G, Laine F, Vedeilhie C et al. A multi-disciplinary approach to treating hepatitis C with interferon and ribavirin in alcohol-dependent patients with ongoing abuse. J Hepatol. 2012;56(2):334–40.

393. Impact of Physician Directed Education on Patient Compliance With Hepatitis C Therapy (OPTIMAL). Chronic Liver Disease Foundation; 2014. (https://clinicaltrials.gov/ct2/show/NCT01405027, accessed 6 February 2017).

394. Compliance of HCV genotype 1 infected patients receiving pegintron/rebetol and a patient assistance program (Study P04671). Merck Sharp & Dohme Corp.; 2007.

395. Adherence in patients receiving pegintron pen/rebetol for hepatitis C in conjunction with a patient assistance program (Study P04281). Merck Sharp & Dohme Corp.; 2009.

396. Adherence in patients receiving pegintron/rebetol for hepatitis C in conjunction with a psychotherapy support program (Study P04252). Merck Sharp & Dohme Corp.; 2009.

397. Renou C LP, Pariente A. Impact of therapeutic education on the outcome of chronic hepatitis C treatment. Hepatology. 2009;50:729A.

398. Zhou K, Fitzpatrick T, Walsh N, Kim JY, Chou R, Lackey M et al. Interventions to optimise the care continuum for chronic viral hepatitis: a systematic review and meta-analyses. Lancet Infect Dis. 2016;16(12):1409–22.

399. Mwai GW, Mburu G, Torpey K, Frost P, Ford N, Seeley J. Role and outcomes of community health workers in HIV care in sub-Saharan Africa: a systematic review. J Int AIDS Soc. 2013;16:18586.

400. Patel V, Weiss HA, Chowdhary N, Naik S, Pednekar S, Chatterjee S et al. Lay health worker led intervention for depressive and anxiety disorders in India: impact on clinical and disability outcomes over 12 months. Br J Psychiatry. 2011;199(6):459–66.

401. Joshi R, Alim M, Kengne AP, Jan S, Maulik PK, Peiris D et al. Task shifting for non-communicable disease management in low and middle income countries – a systematic review. PLoS One. 2014;9(8):e103754.

402. Kredo T, Adeniyi FB, Bateganya M, Pienaar ED. Task shifting from doctors to non-doctors for initiation and maintenance of antiretroviral therapy. Cochrane Database Syst Rev. 2014;(7):CD007331.

403. Glenton C, Colvin CJ, Carlsen B, Swartz A, Lewin S, Noyes J et al. Barriers and facilitators to the implementation of lay health worker programmes to improve access to maternal and child health: qualitative evidence synthesis. Cochrane Database Syst Rev. 2013;(10):CD010414.

404. Mandelblatt JS, Gold K, O'Malley AS, Taylor K, Cagney K, Hopkins JS et al. Breast and cervix cancer screening among multiethnic women: role of age, health, and source of care. Prev Med. 1999;28(4):418–25.

405. Green BB, Wang CY, Anderson ML, Chubak J, Meenan RT, Vernon SW et al. An automated intervention with stepped increases in support to increase uptake of colorectal cancer screening: a randomized trial. Ann Intern Med. 2013;158(5 Pt 1):301–11.

406. Norman J, Walsh NM, Mugavin J, Stoove MA, Kelsall J, Austin K et al. The acceptability and feasibility of peer worker support role in community based HCV treatment for injecting drug users. Harm Reduct J. 2008;5:8.

407. Bossuyt PM, Reitsma JB, Bruns DE, Gatsonis CA, Glasziou PP, Irwig L et al., for the STARD Group. STARD 2015: an updated list of essential items for reporting diagnostic accuracy studies. Clin Chem. 2015;61(12):1446–52.

408. Guidance for post-market surveillance of in vitro diagnostics. Geneva: World Health Organization; 2015 (http://www.who.int/diagnostics_laboratory/postmarket/150210_pms_ivds_guidance.pdf?ua=1, accessed 02 July 2016, accessed 6 February 2017).

409. Laboratory quality management system: handbook. World Health Organization; 2011 (http://www.who.int/ihr/publications/lqms/en/, accessed 6 February 2017).

410. The Alcohol, Smoking and Substance Involvement Screening Test (ASSIST). Manual for use in primary care. Geneva: World Health Organization; 2011 (http://apps.who.int/iris/bitstream/10665/44320/1/9789241599382_eng.pdf, accessed 23 January 2017).

411. Guidance on provider-initiated HIV testing and counselling in health facilities. Geneva: World Health Organization; 2007 (http://apps.who.int/iris/bitstream/10665/43688/1/9789241595568_eng.pdf, accessed 6 February 2017).

412. Systematic screening for active tuberculosis: principles and recommendations. Geneva: World Health Organization; 2013 (http://www.who.int/tb/tbscreening/en/, accessed 6 February 2017).
413. Corneli A, Jarrett NM, Sabue M, Duvall S, Bahati E, Behets F et al. Patient and provider perspectives on implementation models of HIV counseling and testing for patients with TB. Int J Tuberc Lung Dis. 2008;12(3 Suppl 1):79–84.
414. Guidelines for the management of sexually transmitted infections. Geneva: World Health Organization; 2003 (http://apps.who.int/iris/bitstream/10665/42782/1/9241546263_eng.pdf?ua=1, 6 February 2017).
415. Tucker JD, Bien CH, Peeling RW. Point-of-care testing for sexually transmitted infections: recent advances and implications for disease control. Curr Opin Infect Dis. 2013;26(1):73–9.
416. Dukers-Muijrers NH, Niekamp AM, Vergoossen MM, Hoebe CJ. Effectiveness of an opting-out strategy for HIV testing: evaluation of 4 years of standard HIV testing in a STI clinic. Sex Transm Infect. 2009;85(3):226–30.
417. Bruggmann P, Litwin AH. Models of care for the management of hepatitis C virus among people who inject drugs: one size does not fit all. Clin Infect Dis. 2013;57 (Suppl 2):S56–S61.
418. Islam MM, Topp L, Conigrave KM, White A, Reid SE, Grummett S et al. Linkage into specialist hepatitis C treatment services of injecting drug users attending a needle syringe program-based primary healthcare centre. J Subst Abuse Treat. 2012;43(4):440–5.
419. Kresina TF, Lubran R, Clark HW, McCance-Katz EF. Advancing service integration in opioid treatment progams for the care and treatment of hepatitis C infection. Int J Clin Med. 2014;5(3):118–25.
420. HIV indicator conditions: guidance for implementing HIV testing in adults in health care settings. Copenhagen: HIV in Europe; 2012 (http://hiveurope.eu/Portals/0/Guidance.pdf.pdf, accessed 6 February 2017).
421. d'Almeida KW, Kierzek G, de Truchis P, Le Vu S, Pateron D, Renaud B et al. Modest public health impact of nontargeted human immunodeficiency virus screening in 29 emergency departments. Arch Intern Med. 2012;172(1):12–20.
422. Jones L, Bates G, McCoy E, Beynon C, McVeigh J, Bellis M. A systematic review of the effectiveness and cost-effectiveness of interventions aimed at raising awareness and engaging with groups who are at an increased risk of hepatitis B and C infection – final report. Liverpool: NICE; 2012 (https://www.nice.org.uk/guidance/ph43/evidence/evidence-review-2-69062510, accessed 6 February 2017).
423. Jack K, Willott S, Manners J, Varnam MA, Thomson BJ. Clinical trial: a primary-care-based model for the delivery of anti-viral treatment to injecting drug users infected with hepatitis C. Aliment Pharmacol Ther. 2009;29(1):38–45.
424. Grebely J, Knight E, Genoway KA, Viljoen M, Khara M, Elliott D et al. Optimizing assessment and treatment for hepatitis C virus infection in illicit drug users: a novel model incorporating multidisciplinary care and peer support. Eur J Gastroenterol Hepatol. 2010;22(3):270–7.
425. Crawford S, Bath N. Peer support models for people with a history of injecting drug use undertaking assessment and treatment for hepatitis C virus infection. Clin Infect Dis. 2013;57 (Suppl 2):S75–9.
426. Evidence for action: effectiveness of community-based outreach in preventing HIV/AIDS among injecting drug use. Geneva: World Health Organization; 2004 (http://www.who.int/hiv/pub/prev_care/en/evidenceforactionalcommunityfinal.pdf, accessed 6 February 2017).
427. Hermez J, Petrak J, Karkouri M, Riedner G. A review of HIV testing and counseling policies and practices in the Eastern Mediterranean Region. AIDS. 2010;24 (Suppl 2):S25–S32.
428. Corbett EL, Dauya E, Matambo R, Cheung YB, Makamure B, Bassett MT et al. Uptake of workplace HIV counselling and testing: a cluster randomised trial in Zimbabwe. PLoS Med. 2006;3(7):e238.
429. Collier AC, Van der Borght SF, Rinke de Wit T, Richards SC, Feeley FG. A successful workplace program for voluntary counseling and testing and treatment of HIV/AIDS at Heineken, Rwanda. International journal of occupational and environmental health. 2007;13(1):99–106.
430. Charalambous S, Innes C, Muirhead D, Kumaranayake L, Fielding K, Pemba L et al. Evaluation of a workplace HIV treatment programme in South Africa. AIDS. 2007;21 (Suppl 3):S73–8.
431. Counselling and testing children for HIV in South Africa. Lancet. 2013;381(9865):424.
432. Ford N, Swan T, Beyer P, Hirnschall G, Easterbrook P, Wiktor S. Simplification of antiviral hepatitis C virus therapy to support expanded access in resource-limited settings. J Hepatol. 2014;61(1 Suppl):S132–S8.
433. Xia J, Rutherford S, Ma Y, Wu L, Gao S, Chen T et al. Obstacles to the coordination of delivering integrated prenatal HIV, syphilis and hepatitis B testing services in Guangdong: using a needs assessment approach. BMC Health Serv Res. 2015;15:117.
434. Chen CH, Yang PM, Huang GT, Lee HS, Sung JL, Sheu JC. Estimation of seroprevalence of hepatitis B virus and hepatitis C virus in Taiwan from a large-scale survey of free hepatitis screening participants. J Formos Med Assoc. 2007;106(2):148–55.
435. Community health workers: what do we know about them? The state of the evidence on programmes, activities, costs and impact on health outcomes of using community health workers. Geneva: World Health Organization; 2007 (http://www.who.int/hrh/documents/community_health_workers.pdf, accessed 6 February 2017).
436. Lewin SA, Dick J, Pond P, Zwarenstein M, Aja G, van Wyk B et al. Lay health workers in primary and community health care. Cochrane Database Syst Rev. 2005;(1):CD004015.

437. Laurant M, Reeves D, Hermens R, Braspenning J, Grol R, Sibbald B. Substitution of doctors by nurses in primary care. Cochrane Database Syst Rev. 2005;(2):CD001271.
438. Callaghan M, Ford N, Schneider H. A systematic review of task-shifting for HIV treatment and care in Africa. Hum Resour Health. 2010;8:8.
439. Task shifting: global recommendations and guidelines. Geneva: World Health Organization; 2007 (http://www.who.int/healthsystems/task_shifting/en/, accessed 6 February 2017).
440. Optimizing health worker roles to improve access to key maternal and newborn health interventions through task shifting. Geneva: World Health Organization; 2012 (http://apps.who.int/iris/bitstream/10665/77764/1/9789241504843_eng.pdf?ua=1, accessed 6 February 2017).
441. Walensky RP, Reichmann WM, Arbelaez C, Wright E, Katz JN, Seage GR 3rd et al. Counselor- versus provider-based HIV screening in the emergency department: results from the universal screening for HIV infection in the emergency room (USHER) randomized controlled trial. Ann Emerg Med. 2011;58(1 Suppl 1):S126–S132. e4.
442. Champenois K, Le Gall JM, Jacquemin C, Jean S, Martin C, Rios L et al. ANRS-COM'TEST: description of a community-based HIV testing intervention in non-medical settings for men who have sex with men. BMJ Open. 2012;2(2):e000693.
443. Lorente N, Preau M, Vernay-Vaisse C, Mora M, Blanche J, Otis J et al. Expanding access to non-medicalized community-based rapid testing to men who have sex with men: an urgent HIV prevention intervention (the ANRS-DRAG study). PLoS One. 2013;8(4):e61225.
444. Fylkesnes K, Sandoy IF, Jurgensen M, Chipimo PJ, Mwangala S, Michelo C. Strong effects of home-based voluntary HIV counselling and testing on acceptance and equity: a cluster randomised trial in Zambia. Soc Sci Med. 2013;86:9–16.
445. Molesworth AM, Ndhlovu R, Banda E, Saul J, Ngwira B, Glynn JR et al. High accuracy of home-based community rapid HIV testing in rural Malawi. J Acquir Immune Defic Syndr. 2010;55(5):625–30.
446. Bemelmans M, van den Akker T, Ford N, Philips M, Zachariah R, Harries A et al. Providing universal access to antiretroviral therapy in Thyolo, Malawi through task shifting and decentralization of HIV/AIDS care. Trop Med Int Health. 2010;15(12):1413–20.
447. Jackson D, Naik R, Tabana H, Pillay M, Madurai S, Zembe W et al. Quality of home-based rapid HIV testing by community lay counsellors in a rural district of South Africa. J Int AIDS Soc. 2013;16:18744.
448. Iwu EN, Holzemer WL. Task shifting of HIV management from doctors to nurses in Africa: clinical outcomes and evidence on nurse self-efficacy and job satisfaction. AIDS Care. 2014;26(1):42–52.
449. Leon N, Naidoo P, Mathews C, Lewin S, Lombard C. The impact of provider-initiated (opt-out) HIV testing and counseling of patients with sexually transmitted infection in Cape Town, South Africa: a controlled trial. Implement Sci. 2010;5:8.
450. Kanal K, Chou TL, Sovann L, Morikawa Y, Mukoyama Y, Kakimoto K. Evaluation of the proficiency of trained non-laboratory health staffs and laboratory technicians using a rapid and simple HIV antibody test. AIDS Res Ther. 2005;2(1):5.
451. Lloyd AR, Clegg J, Lange J, Stevenson A, Post JJ, Lloyd D et al. Safety and effectiveness of a nurse-led outreach program for assessment and treatment of chronic hepatitis C in the custodial setting. Clin Infect Dis. 2013;56(8):1078–84.
452. Hill WD, Butt G, Alvarez M, Krajden M. Capacity enhancement of hepatitis C virus treatment through integrated, community-based care. Can J Gastroenterol. 2008;22(1):27–32.
453. UNITAID. Hepatitis C medicines and diagnostics in the context of HIV/HCV co-infection: a scoping report. Geneva: World Health Organization; 2013 (http://www.unitaid.eu/images/marketdynamics/publications/Hepatitis-C_October-2013.pdf, accessed 23 January 2017).
454. Pant Pai N, Sharma J, Shivkumar S, Pillay S, Vadnais C, Joseph L et al. Supervised and unsupervised self-testing for HIV in high- and low-risk populations: a systematic review. PLoS Med. 2013;10(4):e1001414.
455. Krause J, Subklew-Sehume F, Kenyon C, Colebunders R. Acceptability of HIV self-testing: a systematic literature review. BMC Public Health. 2013;13:735.
456. Figueroa C, Johnson C, Verster A, Baggaley R. Attitudes and acceptability on HIV aelf-testing among key populations: a literature review. AIDS Behav. 2015;19(11):1949–65.
457. Choko AT, MacPherson P, Webb EL, Willey BA, Feasy H, Sambakunsi R et al. Uptake, accuracy, safety, and linkage into care over two years of promoting annual self-testing for HIV in Blantyre, Malawi: a community-based prospective study. PLoS Med. 2015;12(9):e1001873.
458. HIV/AIDS prevention, care, treatment and support in prison settings: a framework for an effective national response. Vienna: United Nations Office on Drugs and Crime; 2006 (http://www.who.int/hiv/pub/idu/framework_prisons.pdf?ua=1, accessed 6 February 2017).
459. Policy brief. HIV prevention, treatment and care in prisons and other closed settings: a comprehensive package of interventions. Vienna: United Nations Office on Drugs and Crime; 2013 (https://www.unodc.org/documents/hiv-aids/HIV_comprehensive_package_prison_2013_eBook.pdf, accessed 6 February 2017).
460. Grebely J, Bruggmann P, Treloar C, Byrne J, Rhodes T, Dore GJ et al. Expanding access to prevention, care and treatment for hepatitis C virus infection among people who inject drugs. Int J Drug Policy. 2015;26(10):893–8.

461. Integrating collaborative TB and HIV services within a comprehensive package of care for people who inject drugs: consolidated guidelines. Geneva: World Health Organization; 2016 (http://apps.who.int/iris/bitstream/10665/204484/1/9789241510226_eng.pdf?ua=1, accessed 6 February 2017).
462. Benhamou Y, Bochet M, Di Martino V, Charlotte F, Azria F, Coutellier A et al. Liver fibrosis progression in human immunodeficiency virus and hepatitis C virus coinfected patients. The Multivirc Group. Hepatology. 1999;30(4):1054–8.
463. Di Martino V, Rufat P, Boyer N, Renard P, Degos F, Martinot-Peignoux M et al. The influence of human immunodeficiency virus coinfection on chronic hepatitis C in injection drug users: a long-term retrospective cohort study. Hepatology. 2001;34(6):1193–9.
464. Graham CS, Baden LR, Yu E, Mrus JM, Carnie J, Heeren T et al. Influence of human immunodeficiency virus infection on the course of hepatitis C virus infection: a meta-analysis. Clin Infect Dis. 2001;33(4):562–9.
465. Lo Re V 3rd, Kallan MJ, Tate JP, Localio AR, Lim JK, Goetz MB et al. Hepatic decompensation in antiretroviral-treated patients co-infected with HIV and hepatitis C virus compared with hepatitis C virus-monoinfected patients: a cohort study. Ann Intern Med. 2014;160(6):369–79.
466. Ni JD, Xiong YZ, Wang XJ, Xiu LC. Does increased hepatitis B vaccination dose lead to a better immune response in HIV-infected patients than standard dose vaccination: a meta-analysis? Int J STD AIDS. 2013;24(2):117–22.
467. Getahun H, Gunneberg C, Sculier D, Verster A, Raviglione M. Tuberculosis and HIV in people who inject drugs: evidence for action for tuberculosis, HIV, prison and harm reduction services. Curr Opin HIV AIDS. 2012;7(4):345–53.
468. Getahun H, Baddeley A, Raviglione M. Managing tuberculosis in people who use and inject illicit drugs. Bull World Health Organ. 2013;91(2):154–6.
469. Padmapriyadarsini C, Chandrabose J, Victor L, Hanna LE, Arunkumar N, Swaminathan S. Hepatitis B or hepatitis C co-infection in individuals infected with human immunodeficiency virus and effect of anti-tuberculosis drugs on liver function. J Postgrad Med. 2006;52(2):92–6.
470. Liu R, Li Y, Wangen KR, Maitland E, Nicholas S, Wang J. Analysis of hepatitis B vaccination behavior and vaccination willingness among migrant workers from rural China based on protection motivation theory. Hum Vaccin Immunother. 2016;12(5):1155–63.
471. Guidance on couples HIV testing and counselling including antiretroviral therapy for treatment and prevention in serodiscordant couples: recommendations for a public health approach. Geneva: World Health Organization; 2012 (http://apps.who.int/iris/bitstream/10665/44646/1/9789241501972_eng.pdf?ua=1, accessed 6 February 2017).
472. Patton H, Tran TT. Management of hepatitis B during pregnancy. Nat Rev Gastroenterol Hepatol. 2014;11(7):402–9.
473. Celen MK, Mert D, Ay M, Dal T, Kaya S, Yildirim N et al. Efficacy and safety of tenofovir disoproxil fumarate in pregnancy for the prevention of vertical transmission of HBV infection. World J Gastroenterol. 2013;19(48):9377–82.
474. HIV and adolescents: guidance for HIV testing and counseling and care for adolescents living with HIV. Recommendations for a public health approach and consideration for policy-makers and managers. Geneva: World Health Organization; 2013 (http://apps.who.int/iris/bitstream/10665/94334/1/9789241506168_eng.pdf?ua=1, accessed 6 February 2017).